THE WELLNESS TREE

PRAISE FOR THE WELLNESS TREE

"Dr. Will Menninger once said we can learn to be 'weller than well.' Justin O'Brien's book shows how to do just that. It is a simple modern version of ages-old yogic knowledge and exercise that every person can use with immediate results. It shows how to conquer the normal primitive mind-body reaction to stress and bring joy to life."
– ELMER GREEN, PH.D.
Director Emeritus, Center for Applied Psychophysiology
The Menninger Clinic

"Dr. Justin O'Brien's book is a sensible and practical guide to physical, mental and spiritual well being. It is a dynamic program for the achievement of true health."
– DEEPAK CHOPRA, M.D.
Author, *Ageless Body, Timeless Mind; Quantum Healing*

"Wellness medicine is the medicine of the future. This book presents a broad overview of wellness in practical terms that will make it easy for you to start your own program."
– ANDREW WEIL, M.D.
Author, *Health and Healing*
Professor of Medicine, University of Arizona

"Breath is life force. Learning to appreciate this essential force and to use breath consciously is perhaps the fundamental ingredient to health. The information in *The Wellness Tree* provides clear and accurate instruction to readers on how to learn to regulate their breath toward the enhancement of their health."
– CAROLINE MYSS
Author, *The Creation of Health* (with N. Shealy, M.D.)

"T*he Wellness Tree* is a milestone in mind/body/spirit health maintenance. Justin O'Brien works the reader through history, physiology, and spirituality to demonstrate the cause and effect relationships between what we do, say, think, and believe. He passionately invites us to examine the quality of these life experiences and gives us exercises designed to assist us in supporting our natural interconnectedness. *The Wellness Tree* is more than a good read. It is a way of living and believing; it can be a way out of distress, hate, and illness to optimal experiences with trust, love, and health. It's a choice away."
– JEROME HALVERSON, PH.D.
Dean, New College, University of St. Thomas

"This valuable book puts the energy of wellness back into the hands of the people, turning patients into active pursuers of health."
– LARRY BENZA, M.D.
Roxbury Medical Center

THE WELLNESS TREE

THE SIX-STEP PROGRAM FOR
CREATING OPTIMAL WELLNESS

JUSTIN O'BRIEN, PH.D.

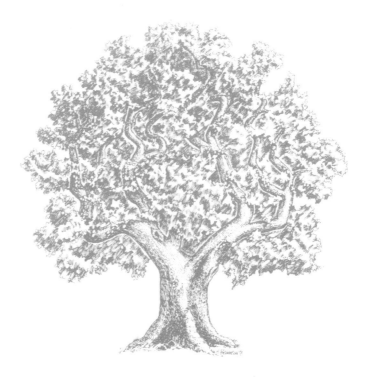

YES INTERNATIONAL PUBLISHERS 🌿 SAINT PAUL, MINNESOTA

Copyright © 1990, 1993, 2000 by Justin O'Brien

Published by YES INTERNATIONAL PUBLISHERS
1317 Summit Avenue, Saint Paul, MN 55105
651-645-6808
www.yespublishers.com

Printed in the United States of America

Library of Congress catalog in the earlier edition as follows:

O'Brien, Justin
The wellness tree: the dynamic six-step program for rejuvenating
Health and creating optimal wellness / Justin O'Brien; forward by
C. Norman Shealy; afterword by Frederick Franck. – (3rd. ed.)

        p.   cm.

Includes bibliographical references and index.

ISBN 0-936663-25-1

1.   Health. 2. Self-care, Health. I. Title.

RA776.O27 1993

613 – dc20   93-10357 CIP

This book is dedicated to
all the teachers in my life
who have led me,
by hook or by crook,
to freedom.

CONTENTS

FOREWORD

MOST PEOPLE DO NOT VALUE wellness until they lose it. During the last three decades there have been repeated attempts by numerous individuals and organizations to promote the concept of wellness: the Kellogg Foundation, the American Holistic Medical Association, the American Holistic Nurses' Association, the Holistic Dental Association, the Association for Humanistic Psychology, Kenneth Pelletier, John Travis, the A.R.E. Clinic, the Shealy Institute, Meadowlark, and John Knowles, late president of the Rockefeller Foundation. All have emphasized the responsibility of the individual for habits, lifestyle, and attitudes which are the foundation for health. Dr. Karl Menninger has talked about the concept of being weller than well. This fits with Abraham Maslow's concept of the self-actualized person.

Those of us interested in wellness as the single most important aspect of life have common philosophies and attitudes about life. These include, above everything else, a positive attitude, a diet that enhances nutrition and is relatively free of junk food, adequate physical exercise, proper rest, periods for self-reflection, productive work, and service to others. These are the keys that Dr. Justin O'Brien uses to promote *The Wellness Tree*, the ultimate in the tree of life.

Reading about wonderful principles, however, will not do you any good unless you practice them. It is our hope that you will heed the very wise advice presented in this book and become truly energized in body, mind, and spirit.

C. NORMAN SHEALY, M.D., PH.D.
Founding President, American Holistic Medical Association
Founder and Director, Holos Institute of Health
Shealy Institute for Comprehensive Health Care

MANY YEARS AGO when I was completing my doctorate in philosophy of consciousness at Nijmegen University in the Netherlands, I felt restless. This feeling surprised me because I had been studying with some of the most astute professors in the world in the fields of philosophy, theology, mythology, psychology, and world religions. But something was missing.

What I didn't realize until later was that I was looking for a holistic concept of life which would bring together the intellectual, emotional, and physical dimensions of myself, a concept that would make sense amidst all the struggles of life.

I returned home to Chicago to resume teaching at Loyola University but did not lose the feeling of restlessness. Then, quite by accident, I met a physician-philosopher-spiritual teacher from the Himalayas who met my unnamed challenge. He not only introduced me to the holistic concept I was seeking, but he embodied that very concept in his person and insisted that the only way to understand it was to practice it in daily life.

So I embarked on a program of self-study and experimentation. I traveled around the globe learning biofeedback, methods of introspection, body work and healing techniques. I researched diets, homeopathy and herbs, practiced breathing and exercise, and studied with unusual people who demonstrated remarkable control over their personal energy.

Reflecting upon all this information, I realized that what was missing in most of our lives was the very holistic perspective into which I had been introduced. This realization pressed itself upon me. While studying Oriental healing and health in Japan, I met Dr. Robert Mendelsohn, an advocate for change in the medical profession. He shared with me his growing criticism of the efficacy of conventional medicine. Then, during the 80's, I was invited to help launch London's Marylebone Holistic Health Centre and join the faculty of the University of London Medical School. There I taught the concepts and practices of wellness to physicians and nurses. Amidst my teaching duties, I counseled patients at the clinic. Most of them had been chronically ill for many years. They had been taking medicines and following professional advice, yet as soon as one symptom departed, a new one took its place. They simply could not get well.

A British survey reported that the average visit to a physician lasted less than seven minutes, so I decided to give the patients the time they wanted. For at least an hour I listened to each person's stories. I taught them self-care practices – everything from diet modifications and stretching exercises to breathing practices, imagery and meditation. I inquired about how committed they were to really getting well. I learned that without 'homework' on themselves, no lasting change would take place. As they practiced, they were surprised that their pain diminished or became manageable; their dependence upon drugs lessened; their flexibility increased; they enjoyed more energy; and they soon became well. As they took charge of their lives, they confessed that wellness is a learning experience that demands a choice and a commitment.

Those committed patients stirred my desire to share this vital knowledge with others. The clients who came after them kindled my pursuit of Neuro-Linguistic Programming and Ericksonian hypnosis, further clarifying for me the emotional and mental framework necessary to initiate change.

The following chapters gather my experiments in living together with ancient traditions and modern discoveries. They present a program for optimal wellness that is simple, expedient, and effective. I welcome all of you who wish to assume responsibility for your wellness destiny and present this book to you.

JOB

APPRECIATION

WHERE DO I START to say thank you? The people, the conversations, the personal stories – so many wonderful, warm, and new have assisted me in preparing this manuscript for publication. Particular gratitude to Frederick Franck for his humorous teasing and his love for community; to the late Dr. Otto Schmitt, one of my mentors in the physical sciences and a playmate in consciousness; and hardly last, to the one who made this all possible: my teacher, Sri Swami Rama of the Himalayas.

PART 1

THE TREE OF LIFE

CHAPTER 1

The Quest for the Tree of Life

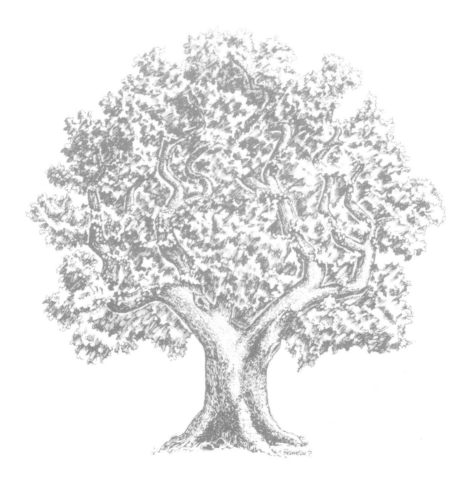

... IN THE MIDDLE OF THE GARDEN
GOD SET THE TREE OF LIFE ...
(GEN. 2:9)

IMAGINE THAT YOU ARE *Johann von Helmont. The year is 1630. You are intrigued by the problem of growth. From where does it come? What gives living things vitality? Where does the energy originate? You decide to conduct an experiment. Carefully you weigh out good black soil as you shovel it into a large, wooden barrel. The soil weighs two hundred pounds. Carefully you weigh a green willow branch — five pounds — and set it into the barrel of soil. Now you watch. For five years you tend the branch: you water it, expose it to air and sunlight, take care that the soil is not disturbed.*

Finally, the five-year experiment is over. The small willow branch is now a mature tree. Anticipating a severe drop in soil weight, you painstakingly dust the soil from the uprooted tree and weight it. The willow weighs 170 pounds, but the soil weighs only two ounces less than its original 200 pounds!

You are astounded. You thought the soil made the tree. Now you are confused. From where did the branch draw its sustenance, its life? You are forced to the conclusion that the life force was in the branch all along. It merely used the resources of soil, air, water, and sunlight to enhance its own life, to expand the material potential that was already within its own self.

In the same way, we human beings are searching for the tree of life, seeking a source for expanding our energy, vitality, and healing, not realizing that we ourselves are that tree. We are alive, we are growing, we are constantly changing; we live in the midst of a universe of energy. Like a tree, we take our sustenance from the earth and from the air. We drink water from the rivers and sky, we transform sunlight into the energy of our bodies. Like a tree, we seek to flourish, we reach out to expand our roots, we extend our branches, we dispense the flowers and fruits of our life force to all those who would gather beneath our unique shade.

Like the branch in Helmont's experiment, we are full of hidden potential for growth and energy, drawing upon the natural resources of our environment to bring ourselves to maturity.

But in the midst of all the riches of the garden some of us appear to wither and fade. Why? We all live well or poorly because of many factors in our environment: the air we breathe, the water we drink, the food we eat, the work we perform, the people with whom we socialize. These factors delight or oppress us, stimulate or bore us. The quality of their existence is vital to ours. One factor, however, stands out as the single most important element for our state of wellness – it is the way we think about ourselves and our possibilities.

Life can yield so much more to us than we can ever imagine.

Life can yield so much more to us than we can ever imagine. Whatever our age or status at any given moment, life presents vast horizons of wellness, happiness, and creativity that stretch far beyond the limits of feelings, thoughts, and memories that preoccupy our minds now. We cannot often guess the outcomes that life holds for us, either individually or in a worldwide context. Who would have suspected the catastrophic political changes erupting in the late 1980s in Eastern Europe? Who would have believed that we could send pictures through the telephone? Who would have thought it possible for dying patients to resort to unorthodox measures like diet change, meditation, and positive thinking in order to affect complete cure? But life is surely made of such abrupt surprises. Growth, change, and the willingness to risk mistakes means that we have the capacity to learn and implement our learnings. Life holds out a challenge to us, an imperative possibility, to draw upon its abundance and energize ourselves into a state of optimum wellness with all its implications.

Promoting optimal wellness means the continuing self-realization of the human potential in body, mind, and spirit. It is the process of actualizing a body that is strong, fit, and pleasurable; a mind that is curious, balanced and reflective and that operates with an ease towards other beings; a spirit that is constantly and mutually self-enriching in its relationships with the cosmos and its inhabitants.

Some decades ago, Donald Schon, a writer in organizational thinking, argued that creativity can often arise from "displacement of concepts." Concepts taken from one field of life and analogously applied to another yield genuinely fresh insights. In like manner, this book proposes to change the common understanding of human beings as well as the way you personally understand yourself by looking at both in a new way.

What if you were totally made of energy? Not just mechanical or electrical energy, but a field of *living* energy. What if your bones, your muscles, your blood, your brain, your thinking were variations of energy with its primary thrust being rejuvenation and the development of ever-increasing self-knowledge. Well, here's the surprise: that is exactly what you are! Your entire embodied being is conscious energy. In fact, energy is the entire universe, and we human beings live in a vast sea of varying energy fields radiating in time and space. Human energy is not classified, however, in the familiar way engineers or physicists would have it. Your energy is a special type of energy that has functions and properties unique to humans alone. Its most outstanding characteristics are that it is self-organizing, self-renewing, self-conscious, and self-transcendent.

Even when you neglect yourself, the fundamental dynamism of your life force struggles towards the promotion of health and retains its potential to carry you beyond the mere absence of disease into progressive wellness. If this were not so, you could not heal your body or exceed conventional knowledge in any area of learning.

You are an energy being. This simple idea is central to the development of optimum wellness, yet it has escaped common understanding as well as medical practice. We have unfortunately restricted our everyday understanding of energy to only a gross, mechanical meaning. In the twentieth century, scientists arrived at the notion that matter is truly condensed energy. From a functional perspective, the energy of your conscious life force forms your body and mind and executes all your functions of living. It also mends your organism whenever that is required. You can, of course, think of yourself either as a self-conscious energy being or as akin to a machine with biological plumbing. Your mind will accept either position. The behavioral consequences of each concept, however, are drastically not the same.

If you conceive of yourself in a mechanical static way, believing that you have only so many years of declining existence, then most likely your body will conform to your decision. Your behavior will match your thinking. Your lifestyle – that malleable, personal complex of ideas, values, relationships and behavior – will reinforce your static conceptual viewpoint, often resulting in a self-fulfilling prophecy. You will live a 'normal' life of failing health, age accordingly, and most likely die of some disease at the appropriate time.

If, on the other hand, you decide not to restrict your vast potential to the limits of a static self-concept, you could examine the subtle energy of your life force and discover that it has an amazing capacity for renewal and growth. Your life will be full of surprises and joy as life engages you and reveals more and more of your potential.

Most of us conceive of our thoughts, feelings, and movements as random, unconnected expressions of our energy. We are not aware that they are all connected to each other in intimate ways. We see ourselves as disparate parts. We do not think that the way we eat affects how we think, that our mood changes the way we walk, that our breathing alters with our thoughts. We don't conceive of ourselves as a network of energy, a unified, whole being. That is why we are not surprised that our physician asks about our serum cholesterol but not about our anger.

THE WELLNESS VISION

So how about a new vision of yourself right now? Ordinarily you take your personal anatomy at face value: weight, color, shape. You feel, see, and think about yourself as physical matter. Set all that aside for the moment. Reconsider your body, emotions, brain, and mind together as an informational network of energy. I do not mean that you have energy at your disposal; I mean that you are self-organized living energy. View your unique power of self-consciousness' intentionality as the force that reforms, adjusts, and amplifies the energy of body and mind. Now recast your feelings, thoughts, and behavior as expressions of your life force. See yourself as an organizational field of energy, taking in positive energy – information – from your environment and sharing energy – information – with those around you.

Some trees grow for centuries. By constantly renewing their energy, the redwood sequoias in California continually mature. Nothing about them is at a standstill; they actively respond to the abundance of life's resources in their environment. In the same context, optimum wellness for human beings is a maturing process in self learning, innate control, and creative living that should never come to a standstill at any stage. More than physical health and fitness, optimum wellness emphasizes a spontaneous and responsible existence that prefers, like the redwoods, to be continually enriched by the acts of living and bearing fruits for others. Even occasional illness or physical handicaps can thus exist within the larger context of wellness.

This book proposes that you can recognize the tree of life in your own being and thus pursue a self-conscious course of choices towards optimum wellness, the flourishing of your spirit. You can, indeed you must, rediscover yourself as a conscious force for the sake of realizing your fullest well-being. The following chapters will show you how to heighten your awareness of yourself as a network of life energy and thus enhance communication between your mind and body for optimum wellness.

This description of ourselves appears strange only because we are constrained by our past education. We are unfamiliar with reinventing the concept of energy and applying it to the entire range of our physical and mental life. But once we allow our mind to adjust to the idea of ourselves from this practical perspective, a host of new possibilities regarding wellness spontaneously arises. When we conceive of ourselves as essentially dynamic organizations of conscious, living energy, subject to high and low levels of its felt presence, then vast changes are truly possible in the quality of our lives.

When we think of ourselves as energy beings we can then decide how energy should flow. When the network of energy flows properly, anticipated positive results occur. When it does not flow properly, problems occur. Place this process into the context of wellness: when your energy flows properly, you feel energetic, you go about life with a sense of well-being, balancing your needs for action and rest. When your energy flows improperly, you are wearied and diseased. You can usually manage to get through the disturbance, but you feel an unspecified sense of imbalance, of being out of sorts, and eventually, reluctantly, you may have to curtail some of your activities.

When you express yourself with and through your body, you are not only using energy, you are also learning through that action what the energy expression means and does to your whole being. It is in the way you understand and use your life's energies that determines how you continue to live from them. You may hate the activity or delight in it. That is part of the meaning of that particular energy expression. That meaning also has a repercussion on you both physically and mentally. If you don't like what you are doing, you will get stressful and tired; if you love your task, the time will fly by and you will feel calmly tired. Either way you feed that "energy as information" into your memory for future use.

Admittedly, climbing stairs, chewing food, moving limbs, thinking itself, all indicate the use of energy. During physical exercise we feel especially its energetic surge and remember that vigorous exercise uses up a lot of energy. While we understand the term "energy" in these uses, we need to get closer to a more accurate meaning of human energy by revising our understanding of its metabolic availability – not only in terms of functional use, but as it applies directly to our rejuvenation. To better understand the living energy network of our physical matter and mental activity, we need to revise the customary rules from describing ourselves as body/mind parts into appreciating ourselves as unified, self-manageable, systemic expressions of physical and mental energy. In this way we can become what we want to be.

PART 2

ROOTS OF WELLNESS

CHAPTER 2

Attitude:
Mind Your Matter

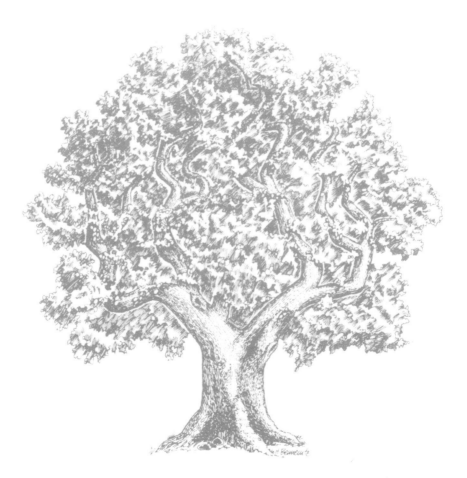

AMONG ALL THE COMPONENTS that we human beings use to respond to life, the most resourceful is the mind. Without the mind we could not become aware of life, be emotionally involved with life, nor take steps to cope with life. The mind is our ultimate resource. By using the word mind I do not restrict it to its rational or discursive function, but include the totality of consciousness. All the resource tools offered in these chapters are messengers of and for the energy of the mind.

The mind is our ultimate resource.

The rational mind makes contact with the external world by using our bodily senses. It also projects its thoughts to the external world through the body. Inventions come about this way. While different minds can arrive at a common agreement about reality, its no surprise that two minds can differ regarding the same situation. Why? Because sense data entering the mind is often filtered through our personal history. Being objective, seeing things as they actually are, is sometimes no easy task.

TO BE OR NOT TO BE

People sometimes view themselves as victims of life. They are convinced that someone "out there" is the cause of all their distress. The enemy, the "stressor," can be another person, event, situation, or even the environment. "That rude clerk ruined my shopping excursion!" "Why did the boss look at me like that? It kept me awake all night." It's easier to blame something out there and thus make myself the victim.

In the movie, *Mystic Pizza*, the heroine unexpectedly spotted her wealthy boyfriend having dinner with a beautiful, young woman at the country club. Incensed by his obvious unfaithful behavior, she angrily dumped barrels of fish into his prized Porsche convertible. Payback! Minutes later she was introduced to her supposed competitor – her boyfriend's sister!

The way you choose to use the energy of your thoughts and emotions is the single most important factor in determining your response to life as well as deciding your physical and mental health. Your response to life is never just a thought; it always involves all the energy of your body. You respond as a whole entity; the entire energy field of your person is affected. The working rule, however, is that your body's reactions take their cue from your mind. The physiological and emotional energy constituting your response complements your state of mind – the judgment – during the situation. The famous neuroscientist, Dr. Candace Pert, remarks: "I like to speculate that what the mind is is the flow of information as it moves among the cells, organs, and systems of the body.... The mind as we experience it is immaterial, yet it has a physical substrate, which is both the body and the brain."[1] Your full response is thus a combination of thought plus emotion plus bodily changes.

Our movie heroine mentioned above witnessed the restaurant scene, felt betrayed in her heart, and vented her rage. In her eyes, her display of anger was justified but, as the evidence bore out later, misplaced. In a flash she perceived the scene, assessed it, and jumped to a fishy conclusion. The crucial question is: From whence did her distress arise? There are always two possible answers to this typical query. Either it came from the facts of the scene or from her *judgment* of the facts of the scene. A close examination of the entire process of personal response shows that judgment played the key role.

YOU CHOOSE YOUR VERSION OF REALITY

Just as we can choose particular foods from a menu, so can we decide which of many possible reactions to foster in coping with life's situations.

Our personal feelings arise more from the way we choose to look at life's situations than from any other single factor. We may not be able to control the weather but we can determine to a great extent how we feel about it. Between the unfoldment of the facts and the way we eventually think and feel about them is the dynamic of the act of judgment. The perception of facts by themselves reveals a certain obviousness about their nature. In our example, the heroine spied two people having dinner. From that factual, perceptual stage she added her thoughtful evaluation about the scene. Out of this evaluation she generated her anger and forthcoming actions. Thus, her mind did not simply absorb the prosaic scene but appraised it. The scene then has a meaning and an additional emotional component that would not be perceived by anyone standing nearby. From that moment on, her corresponding emotions colored the picture to coincide with her judgment.

Without assessment of facts there is no meaning. If I do not determine to some extent what is going on in my life, then, for all practical purposes, very little is actually going on in my life. The discernment of facts requires appraisal; perception yields to judgment. On a shopping spree, your mind does not want to stay in a state of perceptive window browsing; it wants to decide on a purchase.

In many instances, however, the mind has a hard time seeing things clearly. We get used to seeing things in old, familiar ways. The mind forms patterns of judgment based on past experience, which it calls up in similar situations. That saves time. Business as usual. Our previous judgments can thus become a guide for our current perception. This habit also has its disadvantages, however. Take the telephone field inspector, for instance. Whenever he views a forest, even when on vacation, he could see only potential poles. His job prepared him to accept a particular, and very limited, attitude towards nature.

Everyday life is full of situations that can be seen from many vantage points. A new factory is built near the town's picturesque river. To the board of directors of the company, the site is perfect, because the river provides an easy outlet for waste products. Swimmers and mothers judge it differently; they are upset about the probability of dirty water. The town council is pleased to see a new source of tax revenue. Environmentalists tear their hair in frustration.

Events that fall within the gambit of one context are likely appraised for their congruence within that context. It is in this sense that perception/judgment becomes habitual. You form judgments within the context of your job and the way you conduct your daily life. You can not help but form comfortable or uncomfortable energy patterns that bespeak your attitude. You then enter future experiences with these tacit presumptions.

Mr. and Mrs. Wilson entered the bedroom of her dying aunt. For weeks Aunt Rita had hovered near death. She was 87 years old, lovingly cared for by her relatives, and in very little distress. Mrs. Wilson watched the peaceful face of her old aunt and then was astounded by what happened next. The old lady opened her eyes, smiled beautifully at something in the corner, and raised her arms as if to embrace an invisible visitor. Her niece, fearing the worst, frantically called out to her physician husband, "Oh no! Do something!" Quite undisturbed, Aunt Rita slowly lowered her arms and fell asleep, while Mrs. Wilson fell to the ground unconscious. Her blood pressure was taken immediately by her physician husband and read double her norm: 270/160.

Now Mrs. Wilson was taken to the hospital and stayed for a few days. She underwent every conceivable test from blood analysis to brain scan. The verdict was clear: nothing was organically wrong. She was finally discharged with a prescription for hypertension.

Let's take a closer look at what transpired. Why did Mrs. Wilson faint? She had known for months that her aunt was near death. Her aunt showed no sign of pain, was not in evident distress, and, in fact, continued to live for some months after the event. But her niece had a near-fatal "attack" of high blood pressure, sending her body into shock. No one forced Mrs. Wilson to respond in that way as she witnessed her aunt's experience. Her fainting was neither accidental nor the result of a lengthy, reasoned decision. Was her response the only one she could have had? Were the facts of her aunt's behavior so objectively obvious that fainting was the only sympathetic response? It was not a matter of perception on Mrs. Wilson's part that decided her course of action; it was a matter of instant judgment. In a flash, her mind and body executed her personal judgment to the situation. Her husband did not faint; his blood pressure did not rise to pathological heights. He loved the lady, too, but in the midst of the same circumstances, he made a different judgment.

Scenes of emotional intensity evaluated by the mind serve to reveal the intimate flow of energy between mind and body. Mrs. Wilson's body energy concurred with her mind's appraisal of the situation. While the daily prescribed drug restrains Mrs. Wilson's blood pressure from rising so high again, the real issue, unfortunately, is evaded. Although the drug constrains the body systems affecting blood pressure, it leaves the source of the problem unattended. What went on in Mrs. Wilson's mind to prompt her severe response? What continues to haunt her mind?

Intensive and unremitting stress distorts the energy of thought and feeling. When we have the stress of flu, and the body's energy is unbalanced, food loses its appeal. Likewise, when we are emotionally imbalanced with recurring stress, it would be exceptional for our judgments to be clear and sufficiently objective. Emotional stress traumatizes more than the blood vessels.

....

The one you allow to get your goat usually gets your heart as well.

....

Changing one's attitude about one's self, job, people, and the world at large is easier when the constrictions of stress are examined. Without serious reflection on the stressful situations, we overlook exactly what it is that is bothering us. That is why it is helpful to enumerate the factors associated with the situation. Remember, it is not the facts by themselves that stir you but the importance you put upon them. Mere perception provides the data; it does not stir emotions. To evaluate the sensory data means to assert a judgment. Sometimes external, objective dangers that could cause real harm do not arouse a stressful response in you. Why? For the simple reason that you do not appraise the situation as being that dangerous to you. If you appraise it as threatening, your particular emotional and physiological response will prepare you to protect yourself. On the other hand, even if the facts of a situation do not expose you to danger, but for some reason you think they do, your entire mind/body complex will energize a pattern of behavior that characterizes danger.

If I asked you to walk across a plank of wood resting upon the floor, with measurements of one foot wide and twenty feet long, you would saunter across it with casual ease. However, if I raised the plank above the floor, to a height of ten feet or more, your attempt to walk its length would provoke drastic mental and bodily changes very different from those felt in the previous attempt.

It is not how you *perceive* things that counts but how you *appraise* them. The mind decides whether to be at ease or alarmed based on these combined factors. The entire process of apprehending and assessing the facts can occur in milli-seconds, yet after a stressful situation has passed into yesterday, you continue to feel its uncomfortable force by rehearsing it again and again. What else can the mind do? If you relapse into worry, you feel chronically wearisome. The recurring morbid pattern of thought dissipates your energy. The more it assumes a chronic appearance, the more perception ability constricts. The negative pattern stabilizes, and a habitual presumption is born. When this constriction becomes part of your attitude on life, you easily misread people, situations, and yourself.

ATTITUDE AND SELF-IMAGE

Margaret is a high school principal. She continually demonstrates her competence in managing the faculty, scheduling term classes, obtaining grants for the students, dealing with civic leaders and parents, and arbitrating controversial issues with a style that is the envy of politicians. Margaret, however, never thinks she is doing well. She secretly ponders whether she would be better off doing secretarial work. She is superbly competent, yet shows a real – though unwarranted – discrepancy between her proven talent and her own self-image. She easily catches all the "bugs" that "go around" and thinks she must have inherited a weak system. She is not convinced of her value and continues to doubt her future. Margaret has an attitude problem.

Attitude carries the force of your self-image. When you decide that something is worthy or unworthy for you, you also profoundly affect the availability of life's resources for that object or situation. Your attitude espouses the conscious and subliminal energy patterns – your feelings, thoughts, values – that you hold dear about yourself. Your attitude inspires your lifestyle and puts the stamp of approval upon the direction of its energy. It influences your dealings with life and life's potential for you. The importance that you affix to your attitude to life manages your energy flow throughout your mind and body.

....

Your personal attitude frames and guides the energy choices of your feelings, thoughts, and activities.

....

Use follows upon attitude. Too often the central assumption you have about yourself is the firm but impressionable belief that you, like so many others, can not change. On this basis, the pursuit of life is less a question of learning new skills than enduring your fate. Hence, you suppose that a few people may have more and better chances for improved vitality, while most people have fewer and worse chances, and no one has the ability to escape its inexorable decrease as time goes by. The fate of your birth and upbringing sets your limits. What could be more reasonable? You accept the demoralizing assumption that your life force is fixed, supplying you with only an uneven and diminishing return on vitality as you age.

Our attitude about ourselves relates directly to our ability to generate wellness. Over the years we become expert at limiting ourselves. We presume that our energy should decrease and so we notice that we have more and more aches and pains. We start making allowances, seeking corroboration of others in a similar fix. An intriguing question persists: What limits our energy? Is it life itself or is it our attitude about life?

Whether we start from a condition of typical vitality or typical disease, it does not matter: we seem to have the energy that we expect. We may be strong and energetic, old and ailing, or somewhere in between, but if we sense a decline in energy, or have altering periods of moody tiredness, then we feel defeated – at a loss to imagine ourselves in an improved state of wellness. Our discouragement brings our energy down; our expectation is fulfilled.

Transmuting bouts of energy loss and steadily raising your energy level is what might occur if you activated a shift of attitude towards the life force itself. You can indeed get in touch with life's vital power in an easy yet profound way and use it as your abiding wellspring of energy.

Life never remains static. Life is change. Unless your view of life takes daily energy change into consideration, you may become overwhelmed. At the workplace or at home are many opportunities that deplete or enhance your wellness. More often than not, you decide the outcome: your decision reflects your attitude toward yourself. As long as you are convinced that you have the right to access and use all the resources life constantly provides, you can perceive any occasion as an opportunity for growth. If your attitude towards yourself inclines to the assumption that resources for wellness are not available to you, then you place your opportunities for growth and wellness in jeopardy. You won't even see them.

The extent to which you manage change to your advantage is determined by nothing more than your personal attitude of mind towards yourself: your self-image. If you do not want more energy, very likely you will not get more. Life provides you with a sufficient portion of energy for all your activities. You already asked for that much by being born. Ninety-eight percent of newborns are healthy. Will they continue to be healthy as they mature? Will they want and get the same abundant amounts of energy? Or will they opt for less energy as time goes on? It depends eventually on the way they regard themselves.

ANXIETY OF SPIRIT

Many people carry on from day to day with what I refer to as perpetual unease with life – an anxiety of spirit. Hidden beneath their obvious ability to conduct their life in a rational and caring manner towards others, anxiety exerts its invisible burden. Although they would deny it, such people are weary with life.

Carol's house is fairly well-ordered. Bedlam occurs only during holidays. She is sure to always comply with everyone's agenda, but underneath her cheery activity there persists a sense of dullness, a restless dissatisfaction that she finds hard to describe. If she mentions it to anyone, she feels guilty about disclosing her secret. It does not seem that she should be weary, yet she is. So she smothers the feeling with more work, a fuller schedule, additional activities. These choices change nothing except to make her more irritated with herself for not feeling cheery and vital. Carol does not know where to go next.

Weariness of spirit weights upon untold men and women who fail to understand the essence of life. They are intelligent and work hard. They embrace a career, start a family, meet the challenges of living, yet they remain secretly doubtful about life's possibilities for them. The dynamic energy of their early adulthood carries them along – though unevenly – for years. But there comes a point in life when they finally catch up with their unexamined assumptions, that which finally constricts the energy of their growth, wearies their spirits, and robs life of its zest. It is a blessing when that occurs.

Carol has no vision of the abundance of the wholeness of life. She sees life only in terms of pieces of work to be done. Her restrictive attitude keeps the richness of life off limits. She has no sense of a pleasurable integrity of body, mind, and spirit that grows through daily behavioral choices. She has no personal goals for life's expanding possibilities since she disqualifies herself from them. Carol has no joy for living because she does not live from her essence, her real nature: she resists choosing what she really wants in life. In place of a choice she has put a few of society's conventional possibilities and has accepted them as gospel truth although they do not make her happy. She does what her family, friends, neighbors, religion, political party tell her she should do, but she does it without self-conscious, reflective choice. Carol does not know that life itself is a choice, and that everything we do must be choicefully selected. Instead of pursuing abundant vitality through her innate resources, Carol resigns her body and emotions to low energy. She, like so many others, chooses to limit herself and thus smother her spirit's yearning for ever-fresh ways to enhance and express life.

Are you like Carol? Where is the peace that comes from ordering your life around your interests? Where are those moments of surprised excitement that provoke wonder to be shared and a hint of mystery to be explored? Where is that joy that comes from being alone with your imagination in the solitude of your favorite spot? Does your ennui only repeat itself like a weary squirrel on a treadmill? Perhaps you will receive recognition from your labors, but will you also feel the experience of life in abundance? To assimilate just one taste of this abundance can change your entire attitude toward life.

It is never too late to begin. We need only recognize where we are and go from there. We well know how to divide ourselves into time slots and fill in schedules; we are often a marvel of list making to apportion our energy. So why does our fatigue make us suspicious of life? Instead of focusing on the division of life energy into schedules and agendas, what if we consider gathering our energy into a sense of wholeness? I am talking about an idea as well as inducing an experience. You already know the experience of driving yourself into one activity after the other, you already know where pleasing everyone else leads you. Do you also know what the energy of wholeness is like, and where that energy can lead you?

THE DIVIDED SELF

Society divides us into occupations. Tax roles, bank credit, insurance applications, and census forms divide us into categories. Your lawyer views you as a client in terms of litigation. Your physician refers to you as a patient. Your grocer sees you as a consumer who has to eat and drink. Your minister views you as someone who needs salvation. Each sees you from a particular vantage point. Everyone is ready to tell you who you should be for them. Experts tell us how to think about our bodies and minds, estimate our possibilities for illness or recovery, inform us how fast we will deteriorate and how long we should live. The energy of our body, mind, and spirit has been pretty much worked out for us before we reach adulthood. We then view ourselves in light of all these determinations and value ourselves accordingly. We are a divided territory with everyone else staking a claim on our energy. And what is our response to all these authorities? We become conscientious in the endless preoccupation of satisfying everyone's expectations instead of standing back and taking a long, practical look at just what we are doing with our life energy.

Unfortunately, the uncritical acceptance of everyone else's advice for our well-being profoundly inhibits us from enjoying fuller possibilities. Professional determinations are rarely in accord with nature's possibilities. The trends of cultural determinations are not always in the best interest of human life. If they were all true, then we could only go uphill from where we are now. Rushing to accept society's plan for us is not really moving us into a new positive future but merely repeating one weary agenda after another. Following so-called "predictable" rules actually restricts our potential for wellness.

From our culture's tendency to divide things into parts, there is the assumption that your body, mind, and energy are three segregated components. This popular division is reinforced by the proliferation of seemingly authoritative commercials for drugs. Since we have been taught that our body, mind and spirit hardly influence each other, bodily treatments are mechanically induced with little reference to our conscious attitudes or goals.

Viewing our body as matter exclusively, we medicate it rather like a technician tending a machine. Our mind has little to do with this state of affairs except to acquiesce to the assumption that we should be treated like biological machinery. Hence, we presume dependence on external agents for feeling better and for obtaining energy. This approach receives endorsement from most medical professionals. Thus our attitude to illness and the pursuit of health is shaped less by responsible living than by dependence on pharmaceutical agents. If those pills do not bring relief, try these. If that fails, remove the human machine part that is causing the pain.

Aggressive surgery is rampant in the United States. Hysterectomies, for example, are blithely authorized, even without pathological conditions warranting them. By-pass surgery for men is an expensive joke, for the patient invariably returns for another round or two. Instead of eye exercises and diet, we have expensive laser surgery. Along the lines of barbaric medication is the notorious but conventional use of toxic chemicals referred to as "chemotherapy." When the patient gets worse as a result of the use of these noxious substances, that patient is said to have "failed" therapy. The excessive, aggressive attitude of physicians toward chronic disease unfortunately eliminates their comprehension of the merits of self-care and the pursuit of optimal wellness.

Imperative for society's survival is an awareness of its own uncritical assumption toward medication. Relieving pain is laudatory, but many of us mistakenly think health equals medication. The attitude of total reliance on drugs seems to dispense with the necessity of applying the skills of wellness. So the majority of us sit around awaiting illness because we refuse sufficient mental and physical activity to generate optimum wellness. Our naive assumptions prevent us from even thinking about the possibility that we could directly and primarily influence our own energy for healing and wellness.

Here is a typical scenario. You are feeling out of sorts. Joints ache and sleep is fitful. Heartburn surprises you after the evening meal. Early fatigue trails you home from work. Your eyes burn whenever you drive into the city. It takes three cups of coffee before you are fully awake each morning. Finally you bring these complaints to your physician because you want to be rid of them. Physician and patient concur: stop the pain; get rid of the symptoms. But don't bother with causes; don't tell me to change my lifestyle.

"There is something distasteful in the sight of a highly developed society being forced to divert great resources, both financial and intellectual, to the cure of its own self-inflicted diseases. We can characterize these as diseases of choice – those which arise from excesses in its life-style, or the pollution of its environment."[3]

– June Goodfield

Acute infections, surgical accidents and traumas are episodes no one wants in their lives. For these crises we have the emergency room. Too often people assume that their future wellness ought to be guided by what they do not want in their lives. With this evasive attitude, wellness becomes less the abundance of vitality than the avoidance of illness.

With that kind of thinking, helplessness and dependence thrive; self-reliance and creativity diminish. You sense that your future will be filled with fear and irrevocable decline and you desperately look to medication for maintenance and survival. You worry about insurance that may not cover your eventual ailments, or worse still, worry that it might run out. The prevailing mentality of laymen and physicians towards health care is destroying us in body, mind, spirit, and in pocketbook.

Wellness is neither the product of fixing problems nor coping with medical crises. Neither is it about prevention. It does not fit into these typical ways of thinking about well being. The more you try to force the concept of wellness into the conventional understanding of health care the more confusion reigns and the farther you are from its meaning. You have to shift your thinking toward a totally new paradigm. Do not think in terms of negatives (not sick, prevention, absence of illness); think in terms of enlivenment. Optimal wellness is the attitude and the result of continually choosing to enhance your capacity to create yourself anew in body, mind, and spirit.

Optimal wellness proposes that you alone are the artist of your life, the literal creator of your destiny. Your wellness is your mission in life. Why? Because your work, your family, your desires all shape themselves from its energy. If, on the one hand, your mind prefers to think in negative possibilities, then most likely you will reap the obvious results. If, on the other hand, you intelligently access your innate resources in positive application, then you will likewise reap its positive power. Either choice gets results. The secret to growing into optimal wellness lies in knowing how to access its living power. We all possess the dynamic power of the tree of life just by being alive. Life continually invites us to draw upon her for unlimited growth. We can only restrict ourselves by not taking the invitation seriously.

A NEW PARADIGM

Your new paradigm proposes that you are a conscious network of living energy that conceives, draws upon, and governs itself to become its mind, body, and behavior. Change your mind and you change your body. Entertain a thought and you arouse an emotion. It will take some time getting used to the fact that your consciousness

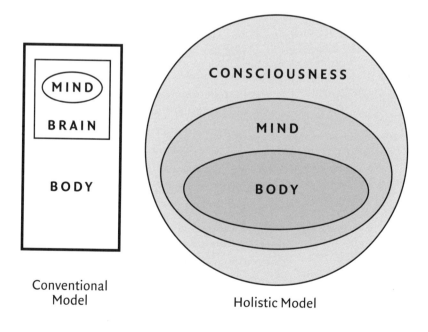

Conventional Model

Holistic Model

goes beyond your brain, beyond the height and width of your body, beyond the limits of your skin. The old paradigm presumed that the brain and the mind were within the body and that consciousness was an epiphenomenon of the workings of the brain. On the contrary, the new paradigm proposes that the body's networking energy, as well as the mind, is within the vastness of the field of consciousness, and only a small but unlimited portion of consciousness is utilized by the body.

The energy you routinely call upon for your current activities cannot be compared to the vast richness of energy constantly available from life's borderless potential. Your immediate horizon of activities, from raising a family to negotiating a new contract, however frustrating or rewarding, is minute compared to the awesome availability of resources to enrich those activities. On any single occasion, you barely draw upon the potential energy of life. Even the simple act of respiration utilizes less than twenty per cent of the oxygen available in your lungs. The lion's share of oxygen energy available for your use remains untouched. Eventually, as you age, you allow even your modest usage to shrink. You curtail your body's capacity to absorb nature's energies, and so your vitality ebbs. Yet it can be reversed.

Why do you do this? Because you think and live in ways that permit only a limited use of energy. Thus you falsely assume that this dwindling portion is all you are entitled to receive. A yogic sage once was asked why people grow old. He replied: "Because they see others do it!"

You have forgotten your inheritance from the Tree of Life. Your thoughts and actions use a modicum of life's healing energy, life's creative energy, life's expansive energy in activities that conform to the constrained lifestyle of your self-image. Your personally-chosen, limited horizon of what you think is available for you becomes a baseline conviction, separating you from the vast bounty of energy at your disposal. Since your mind is set around this self-limited use of energy, you will age consistent with the statistics matching your constrictive knowledge.

With these and similar attitudes, most people slowly suffocate their vitality and force themselves to meet their illness deadlines. They succumb right on predicted schedule. They are like the statistician who contracted stomach cancer and died according to statistical norms for the disease right after he figured out that the averages of recovery were not in his favor. We do this to ourselves repeatedly.

How often do people drag memories that weigh them down into their future? How often do others repeat years and years of remorse or silent recrimination, unable to forgive either themselves or their persecutor? When the mind chooses to remain either victim or victimizer, integrity is lost, and life's energy is programmed to welcome all the degenerative consequences of that role. Too many people face life defensively waiting, for they suspect that sooner or later their well-being may fall into the hands of any knave who chooses to abuse it.

....

"I do not believe that I have excess hostility; this is due in part to the fact that my intellectual, physical, cultural, and hereditary attributes surpass those of 98 percent of the bastards I have to deal with. Furthermore those dome-head fitness freaks, goody-goody types that make up the alleged 2 percent are, no doubt, faggots anyway, whom I could beat out in a second if I weren't so damn busy fighting every minute to keep that 98 percent from trying to walk over me."[5]

– The Healing Brain

....

The attitude that inspires your lifestyle monitors the extent of your energy. If you cannot get seriously stressed, it's unlikely that you can get seriously unwell. If I can produce morbid thoughts that drain my energy, then why can't I produce positive thoughts that enhance my energy? Attitude is all.

Your new paradigm means that you are a conscious field of living energy that conceives, draws upon, and governs itself to become its mind, body, and behavior. For generating abundant vitality you have to orchestrate your energy with skill, love, and bravery, all of which first requires a change of attitude towards your potential wellness. Skill means that you know how to access your innate resources; love means that you have the conviction that you are worthy of them, and bravery means that you continually redefine your lifestyle to live in

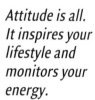

Attitude is all. It inspires your lifestyle and monitors your energy.

accord with the energy of life's abundant possibilities.

Life's abundance is ready for your daily enrollment. Your attitude toward yourself is your first tool for wellness. Choose well.

....

"The best doctors in the world are Doctor Diet, Doctor Quiet, and Doctor Merryman."

– Jonathan Swift

....

PRACTICE SESSION

Progressive Relaxation Exercise

The physical patterns of stress that overload your body very likely hide their identity. You are probably not even aware which muscles you habitually constrict. Muscular tension does not always reveal itself to your rational awareness. You are probably also unaware that stress affects your general fatigue.

Progressive relaxation produces a global effect upon stress. It permits a general release of tension throughout the body which allows for an increase in your awareness of your body. With the release of muscular strain, metabolism improves.

The best posture for progressive relaxation is supine. You may lie on the floor or on your bed, but if you choose a bed, make sure that you are lying on a firm mattress. Loosen up your clothing. Remove your shoes. Turn off your phone. Tone down or eliminate the lighting in the room. Place a small pillow or folded blanket under your head. Take care to ensure a quiet, calm atmosphere.

Your fatigue may become quite evident with your inability to remain awake during progressive relaxation. Do not get into the habit of falling asleep during this practice. If you discover you are too tired to continue, postpone the practice and take a nap instead. You want to remain attentive in order to gain the maximum benefit. Eventually, your practice will pay off by stimulating your inner awareness to be keenly alert to incipient new stress during the day's activities.

- LIE DOWN so that your legs are stretched out and spread about eighteen to twenty-four inches apart. Your arms are about 10 inches away from your sides, with your palms facing upwards.

- CLOSE YOUR EYES and mouth and begin breathing through your nose for ten cycles of exhalation and inhalation. Allow your abdomen to rise with each inhalation and fall with each exhalation.

- NOW BRING YOUR ATTENTION to the flow of your breath. Watch for any jerkiness in the flow and make the flow as smooth as possible.

- BREATHE ten more cycles.

- NOW BRING YOUR INNER ATTENTION to the middle of your forehead and request your entire body to release any tensions, congestion, and stiffness there. Continue to breathe deeply.

- CONTINUE TO BREATHE DEEPLY as you become aware of each body part. Bring your attention slowly down the body in the following sequence:
  eyebrows and eyelids
  cheeks
  jaw
  neck muscles
  shoulders.

- NEXT, MOVE YOUR ATTENTION down your arms to your finger tips. Exhale deeply.

- SLOWLY RETURN YOUR ATTENTION up the arms into the shoulders as you inhale. Breathe deeply.

- NOW MOVE YOUR ATTENTION into your chest. Inhale and exhale deeply two times at the center of your chest.

- BREATHE DEEPLY as you move your attention to each body part as follows:
  solar plexus
  hips
  pelvis
  thighs

calf muscles
ankles
feet and toes.

🍃 NOW BREATHE as though you are exhaling from the crown of your head down your body and out your toes, and inhale from your toes up the body and out through the crown of your head.

🍃 CONTINUE THIS BREATHING for 9 minutes, breathing smoothly and evenly.

🍃 WHEN YOU ARE FINISHED, turn onto your left side and arise slowly to keep your nervous system peaceful.

Tension/Relaxation Exercise

Muscles conform into stress patterns when strain is sustained or when the body is restricted to limited positions while working. To undo the sedentary and restrictive patterns, a systematic process of conscious tension followed by release can re-pattern the flow of energy, induce muscular relaxation, and heighten your body aware-ness. Do not assume that harsh intensity means better fitness; the simplicity of the following exercise overshadows its power. It is a superb practice for restoring and amplifying your body/mind com-munication.

First, prepare yourself by lying down on the floor or a firm bed. Assume the posture of the previous practice. Begin deep breathing for 1–2 minutes allowing the flow of breath to proceed smoothly.

You will now be sequentially extending specific limbs outward, growing them longer, as it were, and holding the extension-tension for 5 seconds. Then release the tension with an exhalation. Between each tension and release is a pause. During this pause in activity, exhale and inhale two times. Concentrate only on each specific body part and let the rest of your body remain at ease.

🍃 EXTEND AND TENSE your right foot and leg as though you were trying to lengthen your leg by pointing your foot.

🍃 RELEASE TENSION. Exhale and inhale twice.

- **EXTEND AND TENSE** your left leg and foot as though you were trying to lengthen your leg by pointing your foot.

- **RELEASE TENSION.** Exhale and inhale twice.

- **EXTEND AND TENSE** your right arm and hand.

- **RELEASE TENSION.** Exhale and inhale twice.

- **EXTEND AND TENSE** your left arm and hand.

- **RELEASE TENSION.** Exhale and inhale twice.

- **EXTEND AND TENSE** together your right leg and foot, and your right arm and hand.

- **RELEASE TENSION.** Exhale and inhale twice.

- **EXTEND AND TENSE** together your left leg and foot, and your left arm and hand.

- **RELEASE TENSION.** Exhale and inhale twice.

- **EXTEND AND TENSE** together your legs and arms.

- **RELEASE TENSION.** Exhale and inhale twice.

- **EXTEND AND TENSE** together your left leg and foot, and your right arm and hand.

- **RELEASE TENSION.** Exhale and inhale twice.

- **EXTEND AND TENSE** together your right leg and foot, and your left arm and hand.

- **RELEASE TENSION.** Exhale and inhale twice.

- **EXTEND AND TENSE** both feet and legs.

- **RELEASE TENSION.** Exhale and inhale twice.

- **EXTEND AND TENSE** both arms and hands.

- **RELEASE TENSION.** Exhale and inhale twice.

- **EXTEND AND TENSE** simultaneously all your limbs and neck-head.

- RELEASE TENSION. Exhale and inhale twice.

- REPEAT THE TENSION in your entire body all at once.

- RELEASE ALL TENSION and breathe until your breath is calm again.

This practice may also be done sitting in a chair. Your concentration will improve as you become accustomed to the practice. Its benefits derive from the complete attention given to each segment of the body, and the release of the tension in conjunction with the breathing.

NOTE: These exercises are available on cassette tape; see *Wellness Tree Tapes* on the order page.

CHAPTER 3

Breath:
The Magic Rhythm

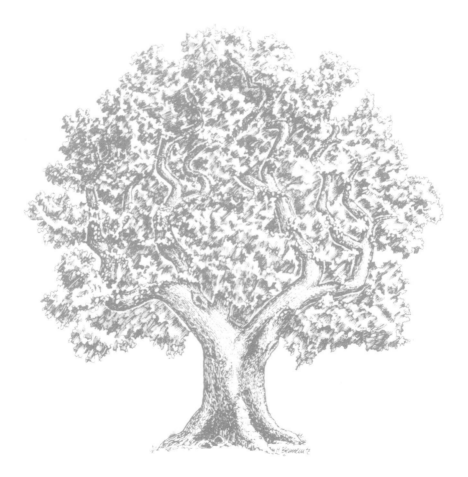

EVERYTHING WE DO IN LIFE is a potential stress-producing event. In fact, it is almost impossible for us to be unaffected. External factors such as the news of the day – inclement weather, an unexpected phone call, a child's illness, a friend's promotion – can all be opportunities for distress as well as for enrichment. Learning how to live a balanced life amidst so many possible and actual stress-provoking conditions demands an awareness well beyond that needed for repairing your VCR. While we do not have to be immediately conscious of all the changes that the body undergoes in order to maintain a balanced internal state, we should increase our alertness to possible stress factors. What we do not know about stress can hurt us.

To deal with life intelligently so that our career and duties enhance, or at least support, our wellness, we need to learn energy-producing strategies that diminish the presence of severe unmanageable conflicts. Without these strategies we remain vulnerable before the whims of our thinking and our environment, not all of which are beneficial. One of the most effective strategies against stress is breathing, as we will see shortly. But first, let's take a look at stress itself.

LIFE AND STRESS

Supposed causes of stress, or what may be called *stressors* are those external factors that are not necessarily under our control, such as the events in our environment and persons we encounter. The variety of stressors is unlimited. While you cannot ever begin to calculate the external factors that could possibly cross your path on any given day, you can learn to manage your responses to them, as we noted in chapter two. Management of emotional response leads to wellness.

I'm sure you've gotten used to reacting in certain emotional ways to your environment, regardless of the cost. You can get things done, get them done well, and on time. Occasionally, you experience moments when your best attempts outstrip your body's reserves to sustain the effort: your will drives ahead but your body drags behind. You pay no great concern to that because when you let up, in spite of your exhaustion, you feel good. Task accomplished. Meanwhile, the frequency of these stressful occasions multiply and you find yourself falling asleep reading the paper or watching television. Headaches soon intervene in your day, patience with others gets shorter, and you reach for drugged relief. In a few days the entire drama repeats itself.

....

"Stress is more than being "up tight" occasionally or having a bad day. It is a recurring imbalance resulting in the daily wear and tear on the body that leads to dysfunction and debilitation. It comes in different guises. Emotional stress (or mental stress) is the stress generated by our personality as we interact with our environment on a day-to-day basis (this is sometimes referred to as social stress). Digestive stress is the stress we get from poor eating habits. Environmental stress is created by such factors as smog, noise and air pollution. The reason stress is harmful is because we are unconsciously creating it, and we become accustomed to sustaining it. Consequently we come to accept stress as a "normal" part of everyday life."[1]

– Phil Nuernberger, Ph.D.
....

The human body is not a biological machine, no matter how much pharmaceutical advertising promotes that medical assumption. Under severe stress we forget that truth. We approach the pain of stress as though our bodies were chemical machines: for headaches, take aspirin; for upset stomachs, Pepto-Bismol; for emotional tension, Darvon; for depression, Prozac; for bodily pain in general, nothing beats Tylenol. Our idea is to suppress by medication that part of the body that hurts. Some people even attempt to anesthetize the brain as a lifestyle. Why not get rid of pain quickly and conveniently? Acute awareness brings distress; therefore, it's off limits.

Over a period of weeks and months, we develop a conscious relationship with our periodic pain that builds mechanical, stressful responses into our lifestyle. What we do becomes habitual, forming its own energy patterns restricting change. Taking occasional pain relievers is not the issue, but incorporating them into our consciousness as a way of living becomes an addiction. We inadvertently use one stress factor, the drug, to suppress another stress factor, the pain. Since all drugs are toxic, they produce their own distress upon the body as they go about their business. Meanwhile we lose the opportunity to learn how to use our stress to upgrade the quality of our life.

DOWNWARD COLLAPSE

In fulfilling tasks that depend upon accessing energy, there is a fine line between fidelity to work and foolishness to self. There are times when your determination to continue working carries you through, regardless of your inability to extend your energy. By sheer willpower alone you meet the personal or business goals you have set for yourself. In spite of abiding fatigue, you call forth seemingly undiminished reserves. In fact, you often use tiredness itself as a private index to prove that you are working invaluably hard. A serious problem exists here even though you can't acknowledge it.

Alas, your mental and physical pace cannot be sufficiently supplied by the energy at your current disposal. You are using up more energy than can be replaced. So you assume that your sincere will to accomplish the task at hand can compensate for the lack of vitality. The more you try to succeed, however, the harder the struggle becomes and the more miserable you feel. Too bad. Lashing your tired self with the whip of willpower becomes a persecution, but the fear of impending defeat, threatening your self-esteem, pushes you on until you are forced to stop.

Battlefield conditions or not, eventually this striving attitude will catch up with you. It will manifest sooner or later in various guises from general irritability, sleeplessness, loss of appetite, and sexual impotence, to chronic exhaustion, anxiety, self-doubt, slipping concentration, and melancholy. Exceedingly rare is the heart attack that comes from exertion at the picnic grounds; one has been setting up the heart for months and years to conclude that painful mission. A homeostatic imbalance of energy intrudes; bodily organs suffer. Society labels it burnout.

The pathetic tragedy is that one thinks life is worth living on these terms!

PHYSIOLOGY OF STRESS

Any thoughtful and emotive response to life is always associated with the physiological changes mediated through the autonomic nervous system. The autonomic nervous system possesses two functional branches: the sympathetic and the parasympathetic. The sympathetic nervous system accelerates bodily functions, allowing for increased activity. The parasympathetic system slows bodily functions, allowing for rest and recuperation.

Prompted by the mind and sparked by neurological signals, any person can undergo a conflict of interest which we have come to label *stress*. Appropriate action is at hand. The endocrine glands become increasingly involved when the mind requires continued action; the nervous discharge is supplemented by hormonal release. The immune system becomes involved since all the energy systems of mind and body act in unison. The immune system, of course, is the body's first protection against illness. When we have little or no

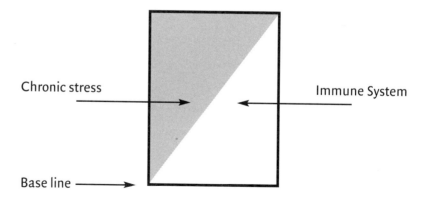

THE WELLNESS TREE

stress, our immune system works at optimal power. As stress accumulates, however, there is a corresponding decrease in the optimal functioning of the immune system. They work together in inverse proportion.

An assumed threat or challenge, for example, demands immediate, responsive action to stir your body. These biological alterations immediately translate into the emotions you feel. Hormonal secretions, pervasively flowing throughout your blood stream, account for the lingering duration of your emotional feeling. The emotional feeling flares up and then lingers even after the situation has passed; what made you angry is over, but you still feel upset. That is because your bloodstream carries the hormonal secretions; your entire network of cells was involved. It takes time for the hormonal chemicals to recede. You had a total-person response. Your eyes were not angry; you were. And if the response continues long enough (or recurs frequently), the weakened immune system will become susceptible to illness.

Of course, not everyone reacts in the same way to the same stimulus. That's why it is hard to name stressors. There is a certain proportion, however, or assessment – highly subjective – between the situation and the body response. While some things bother you they may not bother me or, at least not to the same extent. Leaving the toothpaste uncapped, for example, provokes curious responses from bathroom occupants in the same household. Whenever an emotion is experienced, its duration and intensity will vary remarkably from one individual to another.

In occupations that require a frequent and rapid response to situations – pilots, air traffic controllers, police work, or emergency room personnel, for example – frequent rest is mandatory. Without rest, the body cannot renew itself properly. Constant stimulation of the sympathetic nervous system acts as a restraint upon the body's renewal processes. The smoldering stress of anger or anxiety excites the catabolic hormones which interfere with rest and renewal; adrenaline prevents the cell division that is necessary for healing. When the body gets flooded with intolerable levels of adrenaline, heart cells can die. These pockets of dysfunctional cells then interfere with the normal electrical workings of the heart. The disruptive outcome of such intense activity by the psycho-biology is a profound negative change in the body, both immediate and long term. In a sense, prolong sadness inversely mirrors chronic anger. Unless there is periodic restoration, the person becomes a candidate for self-destruction.[2]

Research indicates, for example, that when high blood pressure is repeatedly sustained for long periods, the body gradually accepts this state of affairs as its norm. An elevated pressure level will then remain abnormally high even when there is no stimulus to provoke it. Hence, the developing history of internal stress establishes a new basal level, and now full relaxation and renewal is out of the question. The body-mind fluctuates in a state of involuntary arousal even though there is nothing around to account for the agitation. Such a person becomes a full-blown stressed state.[3]

....

"If you prolong the stress, by being unable to control it or by making it too potent or long-lived, then the same molecules that mobilized you for the short haul now debilitate your performance."[4]

....

There are situations, on the other hand, that call forth a completely different response to stress. We usually pay so much attention to fierce arousal and frantic escape that the other side of stress imbalance receives scant attention. That side is the stress of sadness. Sometimes people harbor grief and prolonged sadness without showing it. I find this sadness response especially among women, older people, people of color, and those whose lives bear the hidden burden of hopeless resignation.

While the dramatic signs of stressful living are most evident in the "busy-ness syndrome," the vast majority of people suffer stress from lack of sufficient, enlivening enrichment. Poverty, unemployment, domestic tensions, low work morale, diminished self-esteem, occupational boredom, feeling obsolete, lack of purpose, societal prejudices, and loneliness are the greatest challenges to promoting a life of optimum wellness. Anger about life is much easier to cope with than sadness. While in the throes of despondency, most people do not know how to summon their energies. They are helpless when faced with prolonged setbacks that frustrate their creativity and deprive them of enriching experiences. Some reach a stage where life is not worth fighting for. Neither fear nor anger make sense, for they can sustain neither. What's the use? They think that life has nothing to offer them. They don't care, nothing counts, they feel devoid of hope. At its worst, sadness yields a gradual recession from life and thus is most destructive to bodily energies.

The physiological symptoms that emerge with the stress of sadness can surface as combinations of reduction in heart rate and blood pressure, loss of skeletal muscle tone, weakened digestion, and hormonal irregularities. The cognitive and emotional retreat from reality translates into an abiding sense of despondency. Strength ebbs, numbness sets in. It is as if the blazing sun stopped shining.

Here, as in the conflict of anger, the total person is affected, bringing about a profound, deteriorating imbalance. Unresolved anger can provoke a heart attack but sadness kills the spirit.

....

Stress related disorders – diseases of civilization – are the major factors responsible for our rapidly escalating health care costs. Job stress is the major adult problem. 75%–90% of visits to physicians are for stress related disorders. Costs to industry are estimated at 150 billion dollars annually.[5]

....

Emotions are a commanding part of the human spectrum of response to life. They can spur us into action or make us desist. They are involved with all our thoughts, but while they take their cue from thought, emotions exercise a certain autonomy of expression. We can feel certain moods for no apparent reason. In stressful situations, the emotional response intensifies for better or worse. A friendly baseball game arouses emotion and it spills over into creative play. When the play is over, emotions die down, and the crowd moves on. But when you endure a layoff or unjustly lose a promotion at work, your emotions linger. You might brood for weeks; the stress response recurs. Your memory replays the emotional scene, reinforcing energy patterns that sap your vitality. Interestingly, the occurrence of heart dysfunctions increased among normal, healthy mid-thirty-year-old engineers at NASA whenever the current contract ended and forced them into layoffs.

To summarize, we can choose one of four basic responses to stress. First, we may respond with fear, which is the hope to escape from the stressor. Second, we may respond with anger, which is the hope to defeat the stressor. Third, if the situation is judged as so intolerable that both these hopes collapse, the result is profound sadness. There is, however, a fourth response to the stressor. It is magnanimity, the resolute hope to create something meaningful. Rising to the challenge, we exercise boldness; we dare to think magnanimous thoughts. We are convinced of our value and this attitude sustains our innate energy to search for alternatives to pursue our goals.

FOUR RESPONSES TO STRESS

hope to create = bold, magnanimity

▲

hope to escape = fear ◄ **life force** ► hope to defeat = anger

▼

hope collapses = profound sadness

A NEW TOOL

Once you understand the dynamics of energy control, you have at your disposal another tool with which to monitor your mental and emotional response. This profound resource is your breath. Since breathing is both voluntary and involuntary, we can take advantage of this latitude to change habitual emotional patterns.

Your emotions express their specific energy in every part of your cellular energy field. The "feel" of your breathing – deep or shallow, rough or smooth – expresses the energy status of your well being. What comes as a surprise is that your manner of breathing reflects and influences the composition of your thinking and feeling.

Indulge any emotion – anger, sadness, joy or hate – and your breath will change. Your breath is a telltale sign of your state of affairs.

....

"Our breathing reflects every emotional or physical effort and every disturbance. It is also sensitive to the vegetative processes."[6]

– Moshe Feldenkrais

....

The constant vital factor that connects your mind and body is breathing. The way you breathe promotes or demotes the energy of your well-being more than any other single physiological factor. We can say that breathing expresses the vital connection between body, emotions and mind. Breathing is the essential connection and the flow of the connection is the energizing that occurs objectivity and is felt subjectivity. Hence, as you breathe, so goes your embodied life force.

In general, people get along in life by breathing in any manner they can. Shallow breathing, rapid breathing, mouth breathing, and upper chest breathing will all keep you alive, but none of them can benefit you for long. Those ways of breathing create haphazard energy patterns and can only produce haphazard wellness. In a 1962 symposium at the Houston Space Center, Professor Otto Wartburg remarked that when healthy cells cannot breathe normally they pass into a state of fermentation and become cancer cells. Conversely, when proper breathing patterns are utilized, many illnesses can be prevented as well as healed.

This claim to the therapeutic value of breathing and breath patterns often provokes skepticism, even among medical professionals. Its incredible beneficial power usually goes unrecognized. For one thing breathing is inexpensive. But the fact remains that by modifying your breathing patterns you directly influence your level of vitality. The advantage to your health and wellness is the experiential fact that your breathing submits to your voluntary control. You can consciously intervene in your current breath pattern to make it function optimally for you and thus learn to manage your emotional responses.

BREATHING AND EMOTIONS

Emotions produce startling alterations in your breath patterns. When you get excited, your respiratory rate changes from its previous pattern into one that accompanies your new emotional state of mind. Likewise, when you become sad, your breath rate changes accordingly. It is this unique combination of thought plus emotion plus breath rate that shapes metabolism, the energy of your behavior, and your quest for wellness.

Uncontrolled emotions often get in the way of better alternatives. It is hard to conduct life's work when in an unbalanced frame of mind due to an emotional condition. Some people are subject to a wide swing of emotions and are seemingly compelled by them. One must be careful whenever approaching these people, for it is hard to know which of their many moods they may be experiencing. On the other hand, some people feel caught by a single emotion for long periods of time. They may be held by anger, fear, or sadness, and nothing anyone says or does can change their mood. Emotional moods are sometimes so entrenched that alternative, more balanced, behavior seems near to impossible.

The signs and symptoms of either emotional balance or disequilibrium are always reflected in the breath. Knowing this truth gives you a tremendous edge in shaping the energy of your emotions. The moody shifts of emotions, which show up in the irregular patterns of your breathing, do not have to remain chronic. You do not have to volunteer for stressful emotions. You are so composed physiologically and psychologically that the relationship between your emotions and your breath provides leverage for changing the way you feel.

Learning to voluntarily manipulate the energy of your breath means that you can consciously influence your thinking and govern your emotions. Mood always yields to the behest of breathing. When you change your breathing, you change your mental outlook. Your breath always mirrors your mind.

AN EXPERIMENT

Let's conduct an experiment. As you continue to read this chapter, shorten your breath rate so that you are inhaling in short quick spurts. You will be breathing with your upper chest. Sustain this breathing for a full minute. Now note how you think and feel as you continue to read along. Do you feel calmer or anxious?

If you were to adopt this quick, shallow breath pattern for a day at home or work, your physiology, emotional reactions, and mental outlook would be drastically affected. Do you know anyone who breathes this way every day? Do you know people who inhale sharply every few sentences in their speech with someone? Remembering your own brief experience, can you imagine how they must feel all the time? A caution: often these people get upset with the messenger!

Now, deliberately breathe very slowly through your open mouth for three minutes. Observe the changes in your mental and emotional energy. Do you feel energetic or dull?

NATURAL BREATHING

If you continued this type of breathing over a longer period of time, your biology and your personality would adjust in accordance with the revisions of your energy prompted by this breath pattern. Have you ever seen people, particularly children, who have a habit of mouth breathing? How is their state of health? Breathing relates to everything one does or thinks or feels. Breath is the thermometer of life.

Proper breathing has become a lost art. By not taking breathing seriously, we loose its potential benefits. The fact that breathing continues on its own without calling attention to itself does not imply that breathing is functioning for optimum physical and mental health. In most cases, the opposite is true.

Let's take a closer look at the body's design for breathing. The average adult may breathe about 26,000 times a day, that is, 18 times a minute. The less conditioned one is, the more effort one must expend to breathe. The less the lungs are properly utilized, the weaker their condition becomes, affecting the entire person. Your chest houses your remarkable lungs, the essential organs of respiration. These two spongy masses of tissue extend from just above the clavicle bones down to the diaphragm. Together, they fill out the width and height of your thoracic cavity. They are wider in their lower halves than at their tops. Deep fissures divide each lung into lobes; the shorter and broader right lung contains three lobes, while the left lung contains two lobes with the heart nestling in its indentation.

The light, porous texture of the lungs is extremely elastic; hence their capacity for inflation and deflation. The structural connections that allow the air to enter the lungs from the mouth or nose resemble an upside-down tree. The trunk of the tree is your windpipe, or tra-

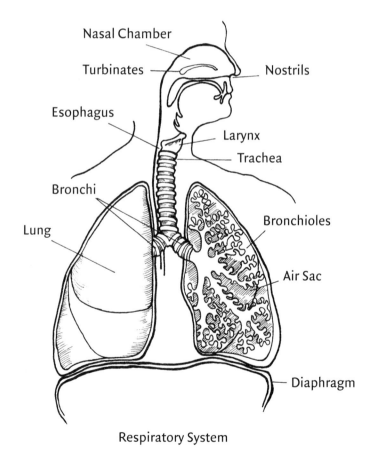

Respiratory System

chea, which extends from the larynx in the throat downward through the chest. The trachea branches out into the lungs, dividing into bronchi, three for the right lobes and two for the left lobes. These bronchi divide again into smaller branches called bronchioles, which sprout the leaves of the tree, the alveoli. In these terminal sites the actual exchange of air and blood takes place.

When we breathe, air enters through our nose or mouth, descending through the windpipe into the far reaches of the alveoli. There the inflation and deflation of the tiny air sacs diffuse new air into the bloodstream exchanging it for the old air. Both airs are rapidly transported throughout the body via the blood by the heart's incessant squeezing movements. The heart sends its venous blood to be freshly oxygenated for rejuvenation and simultaneously sends the newly rejuvenated blood received from the lungs to supply oxygen to all the body's capillaries. This cycle repeats itself thousands of times throughout the day. The bronchial tree services the body with ever-fresh air at inspiration and receives the used carbon dioxide from the venous blood for expiration.

The lungs themselves are basically passive. They cannot expand or compress on their own. They need the assistance of the muscles alongside the ribcage, those of the abdominal region, and especially the diaphragm. The diaphragm is the curved sheath of muscle, acting like a moveable floor-ceiling, separating the lungs and heart from the lower organs. The combined pressure of these three muscle areas against the lungs causes the exchange of gases by the lungs.

THREE BREATHS

We human beings can breathe using any of three different methods: chest breathing, clavicular breathing, and diaphragmatic breathing.

Chest breathing moves the air into the lungs by expanding the upper chest. It fills the middle and upper portion of the lungs while minimizing use of the larger, lower lobes. Since this breathing requires deliberate lifting of the ribcage, often seen in a military posture, it uses more energy than any other types of breathing and causes the heart to work harder.

Clavicular breathing moves the air even higher into the chest and is used for emergencies, when one is winded or utterly exhausted and needs maximum air. It demands a great amount of energy to perform this breathing process and thus is not the normal method of breathing.

Diaphragmatic breathing is the most efficient type of breathing in virtually all circumstances. It employs the maximum use of the diaphragm and is actually the most natural way to breathe. It is the way we breathe when we are unconscious or in deep sleep. It is also the way a baby breathes before it has learned to do otherwise. Proper diaphragmatic breathing allows the richest exchange of oxygenated blood because most of the capillaries are in the lower portion of the lungs.

In diaphragmatic breathing, the diaphragm relaxes upward, compressing the lungs for exhalation of the air. It then tightens and flattens downward, allowing for the recoil of the lungs and the consequent inhalation of fresh air. This basic motion has far more subtle influences upon your nerves, your thoughts, and your emotions than you realize. Stress upsets the coordinated motion between the breath, heart, and lungs. Diaphragmatic breathing recovers the balance.

As we grew up from babyhood, our breathing patterns reflected our adaptation or maladaptation to life. As children and young adults we learned that we should raise and expand the upper chest and hold in the stomach. "Just like soldiers," we were told. Puffing out the chest in order to get more air, however, interferes with the natural rhythm of the respiratory process. Emphasizing the chest forces the ribcage and the diaphragm to work at odds. The constricted abdominal region and expanded upper ribcage producing the puffed chest keep the diaphragm locked upward, more or less unable to descend properly to allow the lungs a fuller refill. It is like speeding up a car with the accelerator while at the same time partially applying the brake.

Whatever the state of your current breathing, however, you can strengthen the diaphragm muscle for greater efficiency and retrieve the basic diaphragmatic movement with practice. As you gradually accustom your nervous system to accept the regulated movement of the diaphragm, you will find that you feel more rested, calm, and in control of yourself even in the midst of a busy work day.

Once you begin to guide your diaphragmatic breathing, the second important modification to good breathing is to pace your breathing cycle into a balanced rhythm. Exhale and inhale with a sense of even distribution of air. A rhythmic exchange of the diaphragmatic motion allows a one-to-one ratio between exhalation and inhalation. Strive for this ratio as the norm and work towards achieving it. The more you habituate this pattern of even exchange, the more you are on your way to establishing the foundational level of your well-being. Diaphragmatic breathing re-balances your metabolic functions. Daily practice energizes your immune system and upgrades the constitutional vitality of your organs for resisting and healing many disorders.[7]

KNOW YOUR NOSE

The principle organ for breathing is your nose, not your mouth. Your nose, together with the connecting internal organs which lead to your windpipe, provides the proper passageway for the air to reach your lungs and for carbon dioxide to be discharged. Your nostrils serve many indispensable purposes for breathing. First, the air rushing over the membranes of the nostrils swirls around to be warmed and moistened before proceeding to the lungs, thus preventing the shock of cold or dry air. Second, the nostril membranes are coated with fine hairs which filter pollution and foreign particles from the air before it enters your lungs. Even before oxygen reaches your brain from your lungs, your nose stimulates brain functions electrically by passing air over your nasal olfactory nerve, directly connected to the brain.

The division of your nose into two nostrils focuses your breathing and your energy all day long. Your breath is prominent in one nostril at a time, alternating periodically from one to the other. This is due to the regular swelling and shrinking of erectile tissue in the nostrils. While the tissue in one nostril swells, the air flow is gradually cut off from that nostril and switched to the opposite nostril. Throughout twenty-four hours, your breath predominates alternately in each nostril in concert with the rhythm of your energy.

Most of the time you are probably not aware that your breath is stronger in one nostril, yet in a healthy adult one nostril is predominant for approximately two hours before the flow of air shifts to the other nostril for another two hours. This natural cycle occurs throughout the day unless interfered with by emotional disturbances, lack of rest, irregular eating patterns, sleep, air pollution, and illness.

This fascinating biological rhythm pulsates throughout the human body, affecting every organ and system, from mental alertness to the healing of wounds. We pay little heed to the crucial work of the breath rhythm though it modulates the basic rest-activity cycles that comprise our daily lives regardless of our genders or occupations. This rhythm of energy is called the ultradian cycle (from *ultradies*, meaning many times per day).[8]

MOODS AND THE ULTRADIAN CYCLE

Nostril dominance is extremely important in any discussion of stress. But as strange as it sounds, the changing of the cycle of nostril dominance also greatly affects your moods. Over the centuries, this phenomenon has been studied by yogis who noted the relationship between the breath flow and its impact upon the body and mind. Among other facts, they found that when the breathing force of the air is stronger in the right nostril, a person feels more active. The converse also holds true. When the force of air flows predominantly through the left nostril, the person desires more passive, receptive activities. Research has concurred that when the right nostril is dominant, the left hemisphere of the brain is more operative; when air flows dominantly through the left nostril, the right hemisphere of the brain is more operative. The entire body cues up for each change.

Practically speaking, your right nostril governs the more dynamic expressions of your energy self. The yogis connected it to the sun because it aids in all active psychological and physiological processes. If one breathes from the right nostril, one feels more energetic, concerned about external work and events. One will also feel physically warmer and sharply aware.

When one breathes from the left nostril, traditionally associated with the moon, the more passive psychological and physiological processes are served. One feels quieter, more concerned with internal thoughts and feelings, intuition, and the physical correlates of thirst and coolness.

Extremes in nostril dominance are also quite possible. Interference in the cycle will prolong the flow in one nostril leading to imbalance. Prolonged breathing from the right nostril can lead to hyperactivity, while prolonged breathing from the left nostril can lead to sadness and apathy.

If you find yourself in one of these extreme moods, you will probably want to get out of it. The easiest way to shift your energy is to shift your breathing. When you are hyperactive and cannot slow down your thinking and actions, your right nostril will be dominant and your left nostril will be almost totally shut down. When you are depressed or withdrawn, your left nostril will be dominant and your right nostril will be almost totally shut down. To get back in balance, you need to open the air flow in the opposite nostril.

Consciously shifting nostril dominance can be accomplished by practicing Alternate Nostril Breathing (an exercise in the practice session of this chapter) for ten to fifteen minutes. By directed breathing you can effectively reshape the flow of your energy and emotions. Another method for shifting nostril dominance is to place pressure on the axial nerve, either by pressing your fist into your armpit, or lying on your side with your head resting on your extended arm. Pressure on the left axial nerve will open your right nostril; pressure on the right axial nerve will open your left nostril.

There are moments when both nostrils flow equally. Usually this brief event occurs during the alteration of dominance from one nostril to another. The subjective feelings then are clarity and poise, with a serene, calm comfort. This middle flow of the breath is the primary doorway to the expansion of consciousness. That is why ancient yoga meditation techniques focus on the breathing so insistently, a fact sadly neglected by most meditation methods. By controlling your breath, you are thus able to control and moderate your emotions, physical energy, and mental clarity. The breathing exercises found at the end of this chapter will assist in the process.

In an intensive coronary care unit of a hospital in Minneapolis, a survey of 153 patients revealed an interesting correlation between breathing and health. It was found that nearly three-quarters of the seriously ill heart patients breathed through their mouths, and all used upper chest breathing as their norm. None of them breathed diaphragmatically.[9]

Breathing properly or improperly summarizes the present state of your well-being and gives a clue to the degree you control your life energy.

Some years ago, a middle-aged gentleman, *vice president of a large oil refinery,* visited my office. He suffered from recurring migraine headaches and insomnia. These headaches invaded his workday two and three times a week, stopping all work and causing excruciating pain. Since he did not want the other company officers to know about his increasing affliction for fear of enforced early retirement, whenever a debilitating headache came on he would unobtrusively leave his office for the rest of the day.

I showed John how to practice diaphragmatic breathing and added a few other modifications. He was to perform these breathing exercises in a concentrated way three times per day for fifteen minutes each time. Eleven days later he telephoned me saying that since he practiced the exercise, he fell asleep every night without prescription drugs — something he had been unable to do in three years. On the three occasions when headaches began during his workday he immediately turned his attention to the breathing practices for ten to fifteen minutes until the pain faded. Six weeks later he called again. As far as he was concerned his insomnia was now history and the much reduced symptoms of migraine appeared less and less. He also mentioned in passing that his symptoms of Parkinson's disease had also unexpectedly disappeared.

Rhythmic breathing induces healing.

Rhythmic breathing induces healing. The rhythmic exchange of inhalation and exhalation not only releases the internal stress of body organs, but the diaphragmatic motion stimulates the lymphatic system to perform its cleansing. Hence, headaches and other pain tend to diminish with regular breath practice.

During the same week, the mayor of a nearby village phoned and told me that he had just suffered a heart attack due to the stress of recent litigation. His blood pressure hovered dangerously at 265/150. Hospital doctors warned him that this situation had to be remedied immediately. Since I had helped his daughter kick her drug habit, he thought I could assist his recovery.

Al was understandably anxious as I instructed him in breathing tactics, first grounding him in diaphragmatic breathing and then advising a certain modification to his breath rate that helps the heart renew its energy. A week later he returned to the hospital for an examination and learned that his blood pressure had stabilized at 140/90. The hospital staff was astonished: never before had they witnessed such a quick reduction in hypertension without any medical intervention. Al was quite pleased by their surprise and told them about his breathing practices. They laughingly refused to consider the possibility of any connection between his breathing and his recovery, and just to be on the safe side, they offered him a prescription for nitroglycerine pills.

Since the energy of breath pervasively connects mind with body, proper breathing invigorates the body and unravels stress patterns in three ways:

- LEARNING TO MOVE the diaphragm so that the lungs contract and expand in a smooth, balanced cycle stabilizes the nervous system and massages the heart, countering its erratic impulses.

- DIAPHRAGMATIC BREATHING disrupts chronic stress patterns, enabling the body's innate healing force to mobilize its energy. Improper breathing impairs the healing dynamism, just as feelings of hostility restrict digestion. When attention is encouraged to shift away from catastrophe, the mind/body communication can return to a dynamic state of resonance.

- DIAPHRAGMATIC BREATHING releases the physical tension associated with emotional stress. The ingress of relaxation instills a tangible sense of self-control over the emotional direction of one's energy.

Breathing will not remove all of life's problems, but the excessive strife accompanying the problems will be dissipated. Life without self-imposed stress is thus possible when one adapts the breathing habits that pace and restore energy throughout the entire day.

NASAL CLEANSING

With so much emphasis on breathing, it is evident that the nose is an important piece of equipment and needs to be kept in good working order. Dust, air pollutants, bacteria, viruses, fungi, and food toxins all effect change in the mucus and mucus membranes of the nasal passages. Usually this change is negative – from stuffy nose to an infection. The mucus keeps these pollutants moving along out the nose, but occasionally there is a breakdown in the system. Irregular lifestyle habits, dry air, poor food, and extremes of temperature dry out the mucus membranes and make them ineffective. When the mucus membranes are unable to do their cleaning work, the result is a rapid multiplication of the unwelcome elements.

One solution to this problem is the use of the nasal wash, or *jal neti* used for centuries in many cultures. It involves washing out the nostrils with warm salt water to dissolve dry mucus, clean the mucus membranes, and free the sinus passageways so they can do their work again. Saline solution is very comfortable to the body; it approximates the composition of our tears. In the nasal wash, a mild saline solution (non-iodized, pure salt) is poured from a spouted vessel into one nostril and then allowed to flow out the other. The procedure is repeated with the opposite nostril. Regular use of this practice will make most sinus problems, colds, asthma, and sinus headaches problems of the past.

BREATHING VERSUS STRESS

Under the impact of accumulated stress, we feel victimized, unable to formulate our energy into a consistent, balanced lifestyle. Since we feel stress so acutely in our minds and bodies, the last place we may think to look for positive resources is our weary selves. But that is exactly where the solution to stress lies – in the dynamics of our body-mind.

I sometimes meet with those who defend, apparently with pride, the valiant conviction that their stress is the result of strenuous problem-solving efforts on their part. They are so stressful because they are working so hard. They are stressed because they hold such an important and essential position in the corporation. Hence to insist that the elementary act of breathing can drastically reverse their stressful condition sounds absurdly farfetched. For them the only negative connection between body and mind is their episodic pain.

Although it is far easier to define stress as an invasive disease, dependent upon the pharmacological rescue of a physician, the self-directed act of breathing is the easiest, most immediate and powerful resource for relief from stress. The strictures of stress vary with each suffering individual but the enrichment of the anabolic benefits of diaphragmatic breathing encompass every real life situation. Regular diaphragmatic breathing enables you to achieve that which in your bouts of frustration and furious effort you are unable to achieve, namely, to take charge of your floundering energy.

In working with your breathing patterns, you immediately discover that changing your breath sequence changes the feeling and tone of energy throughout your mind and body. You also gradually discern that emotional stress and constricted breathing are co-dependent; neither can prevail in your life without the other. Getting through life successfully is a matter of balancing energy rather than producing more effort. As you improve your habit of diaphragmatic breathing it becomes self-evident that stressful patterns of living are as permanent as a summer tan in December.

B – balances metabolism
R – relaxes muscular tension
E – energizes cell life
A – alleviates psychological stress
T – toxicity declines
H – heals body and mind

Because respiration directly affects the autonomic nervous system, proper breathing stimulates the body to strengthen and balance its self-regulating competence. You can voluntarily manipulate the force of your diaphragm and override any erratic breath sequences. The outcome is systemic: with the help of breathing you learn to improve performance in all areas of the body-mind complex without increasing strife. Bodily stress will diminish and your mind will become quieter and clearer.

Various regulated breathing techniques can be deployed for

unspecified ill-health, hypertension, cardiac dysfunction, lassitude, fatigue, and a host of emotional tensions.

The calming relaxation induced by regulated breathing reestablishes emotional equilibrium and frees more energy for the tasks of healing and meaningful living. After reviewing research in the area of self-induced healing with breathing cycles, psychologist Ernest Rossi acknowledged breathing's profound efficacy. He concluded that we heal most readily when we are in a comfortable state. With regulated breathing, ease replaces disease.[10]

Breathing properly has an additional effect on the energy of mind and body because it improves your awareness of your changing internal states. To put it simply, learning to breathe enables you to control, direct, and alter your moods, reversing the dissipation of stress. Ways of breathing are ways of being.

"Breathing is according to the freedom of life."[11]

— Emmanuel Swedenborg

PRACTICE SESSION

Diaphragmatic Breathing Exercise

Take precautions so that the phone, doorbell or other noises do not disturb you during this practice. Loosen your belt and your collar button so that nothing binds you tightly. Lie down on a flat, firm surface, such as your carpeted floor. Place a small pillow or rolled blanket under your head. Allow your legs to spread apart like the letter A. Your arms should be about ten inches away from your body, palms upward. Gently close your eyes.

BRING YOUR ATTENTION to the breathing motion already in progress in the lower region of your chest. Concentrate your attention on the space between your navel and sternum. Place your right hand on that area. Let gravity help this region of your anatomy collapse downwards as you exhale and rise when you inhale fresh air.

- PLACE YOUR LEFT HAND on your upper chest. You should feel no movement here; your left hand should not rise and fall with the breath.

- KEEP YOUR HANDS IN PLACE and get used to the feeling of the movement for a few minutes. Right hand moves; left hand is still. Think of your lower chest as a balloon filling with air and then flattening as the air is released.

- NOW PUT MORE EMPHASIS on your downward stroke – the exhalation – pressing down to get rid of the stale air. Do not force fresh air into your lungs at the inhalation. Merely allow the upward rising of your abdomen to occur without effort. Practice this movement for twenty breaths.

- WHEN THE DIAPHRAGMATIC MOVEMENT seems easy and comfortable, bring your attention to the flow of your breath. Just be aware of your breathing. Notice the flow. If you sense that the flow is jerky, smooth it out. If you sense the flow is halting or there are long gaps during the breath cycle, allow the flow to be as continuous as possible, exhalation followed by inhalation, one right after the other.

- FINALLY, HAVE A SENSE that your breathing is moving towards an even rhythmic exchange. Do not rush the cycle. Allow your mind to coast along with the breath. In this way your breathing and your attention unite for optimum energizing.

Ten minutes of this practice daily will strengthen your nervous system and dissipate stress.

Alternate Nostril Breathing

During the day when you have been working hard, you may accumulate stressful feelings that distort your judgment and make you tense. Rebalancing emotional energy and clearing the mind is important for your performance. One of the easiest ways to clear and balance your system and regain a sense of self-control over your energies is through alternate nostril breathing.

By directing the flow of your breath alternately in each nostril, you allow thought, emotion, and the autonomic nervous system to establish their synchronistic relationship, reestablishing a self-directing center in your energy. Just as diaphragmatic breathing re-establishes rest and relaxation, so alternate nostril breathing reestablishes control over your emotions.

- SIT COMFORTABLY with your head, neck and trunk erect. Keep both feet flat on the floor, loosen your belt. Close your mouth and your eyes. Begin focusing your attention on diaphragmatic breathing. Breathe diaphragmatically for five complete breaths.

- BRING YOUR HAND up to your face and gently close your right nostril with your thumb. Exhale slowly through your left nostril. As you complete your exhalation, gently close your left nostril with your ring finger, simultaneously releasing your thumb to open the right nostril. Inhale slowly through the right nostril. Repeat the process from the beginning twice more.

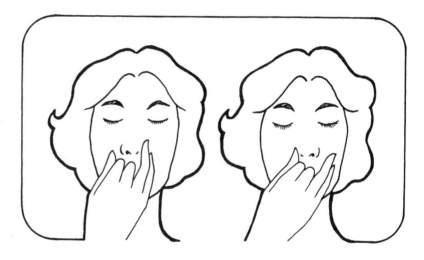

- AFTER YOUR THIRD INHALATION, do not close the right nostril. Keep it open and immediately exhale slowly from it while holding the left nostril closed. Then open the left nostril for the inhalation while closing the right nostril. Repeat this procedure twice more.

- BRING YOUR HAND away and breathe diaphragmatically through both nostrils for five breaths.

🖋 REPEAT THE ENTIRE SEQUENCE once more.

At first, the switching of nostrils may seem awkward. With practice, however, this movement becomes smoother and easier. For some time your exhalation may be longer or shorter than your inhalation. As you become more comfortable with the practice, guide your breathing so that your exhalation/inhalation cycles become more even and balanced. Remember, the diaphragm does the work; allow the breath exchange to be guided by the movement of the diaphragm. Do not aimlessly manipulate your nostrils but concentrate carefully on feeling the flow of the breath.

Cleansing Breath Exercise

During the day, your mind is frequently interrupted. These momentary interruptions, and the resulting pauses in your breath cycle, allow carbon dioxide to accumulate in your body. It irritates your nervous system and produces a general feeling of fatigue in your body and distraction in your mind. The cleansing breath is a powerful practice designed to remove toxins and restore metabolic balance.

🖋 SIT COMFORTABLY ERECT with both feet on the floor.

🖋 BEGIN BREATHING DIAPHRAGMATICALLY, then vigorously and quickly push your abdominal muscles inward as you exhale the air through your nose. The quick expulsion makes a rushing sound through the nostrils, as though you were blowing your nose. Do not hold the contraction inward but release it naturally. The movement resembles a snapping motion with the force on the exhalation.

🖋 IMMEDIATELY ALLOW the abdomen to expand without force by inhaling naturally.

🖋 REPEAT THIS PROCEDURE five times in quick succession; then breathe normally for five breaths. Follow with five more cleansing breaths.

This breathing practice puts stimulating pressure upon your inner organs. Allow a few weeks of practice in order to condition your lungs and increase endurance. Practice daily and every few days increase the number of breaths in each sequence. You should get to the point where you can perform the exercise for five minutes without feeling any strain.

Whenever you begin to feel depleted in energy from the rush of the day, rejuvenate your energy with this breathing exercise. The more you use it, the easier it becomes.

Full Breath Exercise

The Full Breath is designed to reduce stressful constriction in the chest. By breathing as deeply as possible, using the entire area from diaphragm to clavicle, you also cleanse your blood and energize the body. It is a great tonic for starting the day.

- STAND FIRMLY on both feet, before an open window if possible. Hold your head up and look straight ahead. Exhale as deeply as possible, pressing the abdomen towards the spine.

- INHALE AS THOUGH you were inhaling from the bottom of your spine, forcing your trunk to expand slowly upwards like an ever-enlarging balloon. Keep forcing the air into your lungs until you feel your back expanding and then the pressure rising up to the clavicle at the base of your neck.

- ONCE YOU ARE HOLDING your full quota of air, reverse the process and exhale all the air by contracting you abdominal muscles. Feel as if you are exhaling from the top of your neck downwards to the bottom of your spine.

- REPEAT THE CYCLE three to five times. Notice that you may feel a bit dizzy. As your nervous system gets accustomed to processing the increased oxygen, the dizziness will stop.

- MAKE SURE YOU BREATHE through your nostrils. Breathe as smoothly and as rhythmically as possible. Your breathing may be audible at the beginning, but later, when you have more control over the exercise, your breathing should be silent.

- YOUR ABILITY TO PERFORM this exercise increases with practice. You can expand the repetitions gradually from five to ten. After a week there should be no strain in its performance.

NOTE: These exercises are available on the audio *Wellness Tree Tapes.* A small porcelain pot for *jal neti* is also available from Yes International Publishers. See order page.

CHAPTER 4

Nutrition:
Food for Thought

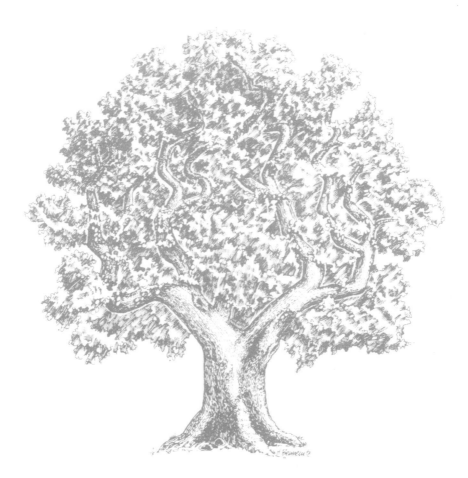

W HY DO YOU EAT? To satisfy hunger? To relieve boredom or loneliness? To experience pleasure? To increase strength and muscle? To become creative and feel well? Nothing else to do? Why you eat is a critical question. Your reply to the question depends upon the current priorities in your life, but it will influence your future health and well-being.

Whatever your reason for eating, one inexorable fact remains: energy derived from food becomes your body, influences your mind, and colors your emotions. Whether you are seriously interested in nutrition or not, the result on your health is the same. You get sick less from a lack of food than from the increased susceptibility and low energy caused by a deficient diet.

Along with proper breathing, the most important source of your energy is food. More than contributing the material energy of your body, food serves the development of your entire person, your thinking, reasoning, and feeling.

Since you are concerned about optimum energy you must also be concerned about the food you consume. Even a cursory investigation into the composition of food will give a clue to its energy potential. The human body cannot assimilate artificial ingredients. It has an affinity only for natural elements. Since we live in a time-centered society that demands efficiency, ease of preparation, and instant results, food manufacturers promote their products on this compelling basis. There is even an advertising axiom used by fast-food chains: they don't sell food; they sell courtesy, convenience and speed. If you approach nutrition from this perspective you can forget about wellness.

The more you select food that contains preservatives, additives, colorings, stabilizers, and synthetic materials, the more you subject your body to energy stressors and depletion. Artificial food products disturb the functioning of your metabolism, weaken your constitution, and interfere with your ability to think, plan, and enjoy life. Ingesting chemicals as a steady diet degenerates the body. In my judgment this is a major factor in senility and disease. The more food is removed from its natural state, the less energy it will provide, and the more likely you will be malnourished.

WHY YOU EAT

Habits of eating are not the same as habits of nutrition. Habits of eating are learned from youth and are thus hard to alter. When we are young – and parents can well attest to this truth – our body can ingest just about anything. We grew up on the four basic food groups, prescribed by the national food authorities, which listed in order in importance: meat, milk, fruits/vegetables, and grain. This was a national campaign for all children and adults and accepted unquestionably.

Like little goats, children consume anything that looks appealing, whether or not it insures proper dietary balance. Snack foods become meals and junk meals become habits. As long as the selection has sufficient sugar, fat, and salt it's fine. Soon children grow into adulthood with an easy reliance upon processed foods, diet colas, vending machine selections, fast-food restaurants, packaged snacks, and the inevitably resulting crash diets. This style of eating fits with the rest of the fast-moving lifestyles in our hi-tech culture. Food advertising does more than support this culture; it accentuates haste while depleting nutrition. "With our convenience foods so abundant," they ask, "why bother with 'old fashioned' foods that require preparation?"

Choosing healthy, nutritious foods and preparing them well is actually a simple thing. But this fact gets obscured in the midst of our busy schedules. The dedication with which we pursue our ambitions leaves no time for a careful consideration of the kinds and amounts of foods that are best for us. Composing our menu is meant to be a delicious pastime, subject to modifications according to season, ability, and mood. The management of personal nutrition should relate to our activities and our individual constitution. We are in trouble if we serve construction-worker meals to a desk-bound accountant, or if we measure our menu at fifty by what we consumed at twenty.

While we are young we eat for our whims; to be creative we have to eat for our minds. In our urgency to satisfy hunger, we often neglect the fact that the quality of the food we assimilate influences the quality of our cells, and thus influences our thought processes. We forget that nutrition plays a profound role in affecting consciousness. Through digestion and assimilation, your body reorganizes the energy of nutrition into a higher level – your living body. You have the power to transform the energy of food into living, human energy.

Nutritional energy also nourishes the brain and nervous system for performing the higher forces of thought, will, and creativity. When your food is fresh, nutritious, and carefully prepared, you feel light, energetic, positive, ready to work. The energy of the sunlight, of the air, of the earth, is transferred through fresh foods into your body. It then becomes your cells, helping you move, think, play, and work.

When food is deficient in some way – artificial, contaminated, burned, too greasy, too starchy, too salty, too spicy – you experience the loss as low energy. When the body is satiated with a heavy meal, the mood is also ponderous. Too much food is recognizably discouraging to subtle, mental reflections, and, of course, physical activity. On a full stomach, it is much easier to hit the couch than the computer. How creative did you feel after your last Thanksgiving Day feast?

TARGET YOUR NUTRITION

The guiding rule: your decision on what to eat should be decided by what you want to do with your body and mind. Your menu should fit the purpose of your life. Whatever food you choose must nutritionally support your overall life plan.

In order to function optimally, the human body needs a sizable combination of ingredients. The customary list of proteins, complex carbohydrates, oils, water, vitamins, minerals, and fiber build the functional matter of the body. From these basic nutrients the body makes itself over and over again. Since the body is always replacing its dying cells, it looks basically to protein for its supply of raw materials. For its energy, however, the body prefers to use complex carbohydrates and fats, although it can use proteins as a reluctant, secondary selection.

Swedish studies of 1967 have shown that neither a predominantly protein diet nor a fat-rich diet contribute significantly to endurance. The ideal, which interestingly matches the diet of some of the longest surviving cultures of the world, is a diet in which complex carbohydrates, rather than protein or fat, are the mainstay. In his book *Holistic Health,* yoga master Swami Rama brings to light some of the proven dietary practices of the East:

....

"As described in the ancient manuals, food falls into two different categories: cleansers and nourishers. Fruits have more cleansing value, while vegetables, grains, legumes, and dairy products have more nourishing value. One should include both types of foods in the diet every day. There should be a balance between solids and liquids. For most this means a diet that consists of about 40% whole grains, 20% beans, 20% vegetables, 15% fruits and raw vegetable salads and 5% dairy products. During the winter one should eat less fruit because fruit makes one feel cooler. In the summer more fruit and raw vegetables should be taken and the quantity of whole grains should be reduced. In this way one maintains a proper balance."[1]

....

These recommendations should be used as guides in studying your own dietary needs. Use a combination of expert advice and self-experimentation in setting up your own diet. There is no one diet that is exactly right for everyone. Some constitutions are allergic to certain otherwise nutritious foods; some bodies perform better with a particular food combination. Hence the reason for experimentation.

Eating wholesome foods should always be your guide regardless of diet preferences, but there are some definite advantages to increasing plant foods in your diet. They digest more easily than meat dishes, giving you a lighter feeling. The nutritional values of plants are generally more balanced and higher in carbohydrate energy than meat. As we have seen, carbohydrates are most important to get us through the day.

Until this century the typical American diet was more comparable to vegetarianism than anything else. Meat was eaten infrequently and then usually in small amounts. In recent decades, the consumption of meat has become more an international symbol of affluence than a sign of improved nutrition. Studies of societies under sudden dietary restrictions, British citizens during World War II, for example, indicate vastly improved health as a result of their virtually meatless, low-sugar, low-fat diets.

The ample variety of foods available today allows for a wide selection of alternates to any diet. In order to know which foods are best for you, study the way your food affects your mood, your energy for work and play, and your general health. Be honest in your experimentation and select foods for the way they make you feel, rather than for the way they taste. What we eat, how much we eat, and how we eat create nutritional moods. A poor diet sabotages our life's work; poor nutrition lowers the energy for our ambitions.

Eventually, it becomes more difficult for us to perform our actions and our goals may even be forgotten.

FOOD FOR HEALTH

In a hospital ward of 450 patients a few decades ago, Max Gerson, M.D. managed to cure all but four patients of the "incurable" disease of skin tuberculosis. How did he do it? He slightly modified their diet. Small nutritional changes, in the simplest way, allowed their innate life force to affect their healing dynamisms.[2]

In 1976 the U.S. Senate Select Committee on Nutrition and Human Needs produced a report entitled *Nutrition and Health: An Evaluation of Nutritional Surveillance in the United States.* The report identified five of the ten major causes of death as diet-related. It further indicated the discrepancies between an optimal balanced diet and the actual consumption of fat, protein and carbohydrates by Americans. The American Medical Association responded to this amazing report by saying there was no proof that nutrition has any effect on disease. Yet in 1985 the National Cancer Institute released a report that at least 35% of cancer incidents related to diet.

In 1991, a momentous event took place by some nutritionists and physicians. Country-wide announcements broadcast the establishment of an entirely new four food group plan to guide Americans to better choices for health. The new proposal emphasized whole grains, legumes, vegetables, and fruits. Meat and milk, which were the mainstay of the earlier food groups, now were considered optional. Why? Because medical studies clearly show that meat and milk are not necessary for human health. Even though the meat industry called its own press conference to counteract the announcement, the new recommendations prevailed.

Neal Bernard, M.D., the president of the Physicians Committee for Responsible Medicine (PCRM) who sponsored the announcement of the new food groups, stated:

"Research is now clear and sufficient that the basic dietary guidelines taught to us as schoolchildren are wrong. Based on the knowledge we have today, we cannot go on recommending a diet based on the old four food groups ... most people who eat according to the old food groups die earlier and have a greater risk of serious illness than those who eat differently."[3]

Later in the same year, in an address before the First National Conference on the Elimination of Coronary Artery Disease, Dr. T. Colin Campbell exclaimed:

"We, as scientists, can no longer take the attitude that the public cannot benefit from information they are not ready for.... We must have the integrity to tell them the truth and let them decide what to do with it. We must tell them that a diet of roots, stems, seeds, flowers, fruits, and leaves is the healthiest diet, and the only diet we can promote, endorse, and recommend."[4]

In 1992 the United States Department of Agriculture finally announced the new pyramid of food groups. Meat and dairy groups were set at the narrow top of the pyramid. This meant that animal products are higher on the food chain and ought to occupy a small place in the human diet. Unfortunately, this was a small step for school children who will still be instructed to eat two or three servings from the meat group and two or three servings from the milk group daily. One must remember that the food groups were developed by the Department of Agriculture and not the Department of Health and Human Services. The Department of Agriculture's mission is to sell food products, not promote public health. Furthermore, Congress encouraged the USDA to increase the demand for meat and dairy products.

The meat industry is about on a par with the American Medical Association when it comes to appreciating the importance of nutrition. An unorthodox medical study was carefully monitored among forty-eight people suffering from serious heart disease. Twenty patients followed the American Heart Association dietary regime which included reducing their ingestion of fat and cholesterol, performing modest exercise and not smoking. The other twenty-eight embraced a wellness lifestyle. They met regularly and exercised, ate a vegetarian diet, did daily stretches and relaxation techniques, and ingested no caffeine or tobacco. At the end of the year both groups were tested against their beginning assessments. The majority following the American Heart Program worsened: chest pains in the group increased 165%, and heart arterial blockages corroded more, making heart attacks more imminent.

The comparison was shockingly unexpected. 82% produced a medically impossible reversal of their arterial blockages and chest pains reduced by 91%. When body, mind, and spirit are integrated, wonders can flourish.[5]

....

We have reached the point where nutrition, or the lack or the excess or the quality of it, may be the nation's number-one public health problem.... we face the more subtle, but also more deadly, reality of millions of Americans loading their stomachs with food which is likely to make them obese, to give them high blood pressure, to induce heart disease, diabetes, and cancer – in short, to kill them over the long term.[6]

– United States Senate

....

In order to improve your constitutional vitality, you must resort to the energy of natural resources. When you eat an apple, its moist, fibrous energy is processed into an entirely different energy form. Under the impact of heat, a hard, inedible soybean is rendered palpable for human consumption. Both forms of natural, living energy are assimilated into your energy field and converted into the living energy of body tissue. We trust the life force to perform this amazing transformation.

Energy conversions are not arbitrary. The processing and dispersion of food follows an orderly pattern, and yet the activity is not overseen by our rational awareness. The discursive mind can be preoccupied with all sorts of ideas while other parts of the body carry out the digestive process. The rational mind does not dispatch instructions to the digestive organs. In other words, we do not command, "Digest, digest!" in order for our digestion to occur.

The guidance of consciousness in digestion operates from a different mode of awareness. The conversion and integration of the nutritious energy of matter from one form into another reveals the positive transformation enacted by the unconscious level of your life force. When we have a good meal in the right mood we cannot help but look and feel better.

STRESS DIETS

During periods of stress, the body utilizes its reserves of certain important vitamins as it attempts to preserve health. Vitamins C, E, and the B group, which are necessary for the functioning of the nervous and endocrine systems, are used rapidly in the body's efforts to survive stressful responses. During these uncomfortable periods, many of us are inclined to indulge in what we consider comforting or energizing foods. These may be foods that mother used to make when we were ill, or perhaps foods that pamper us and make us feel special. Often restaurant food is comfort food for many stressed cooks. Many of these "comfort" foods, however, impair health. Some ingredients – caffeine, for example – immediately stimulate the sympathetic nervous system, activating an inner stress response. Others – refined sugar, for example – can effect a condition of fatigue, nervousness, forgetfulness, and irritability that will lower the body/mind tolerance to pressures of daily living.

SUGAR IS SWEET POISON

Sugar is known as the "white death."

When you use sweets as a source of quick energy, you are working against yourself. The sugar found in candy, cake, cookies, sodas and other sweet foods is easily and quickly absorbed by the body. It renders a quick flush of energy. But we are not aware of the extra work going on in our bodies just to keep us in healthy balance after the effect of the sugar. Sugar is known as the "white death."

Our body's chemical makeup is so precisely balanced that whatever we put into the body has the potential to drastically affect that balance. In terms of emotions and energy, the amount of glucose in the blood must balance with the amount of blood oxygen for maximum efficiency. Our adrenal glands maintain this balance with fine precision. Blood sugar, called glucose, is an essential element in the human bloodstream. It is found, usually with other sugars, in fruits and vegetables. It is the key ingredient in our metabolism, and is supplied by many of our principal foods. Sucrose, on the other hand, is sugar made from the sugar cane and the sugar beet, and in the history of humanity, is a relatively new addition to the items ingested in the diet.

When we eat refined sugar (sucrose), it passes directly into the intestines where it is absorbed into the blood. This new addition of the glucose-similar substance drastically increases the amount of sugar, upsetting the balance. We become tired, listless, irritable, nervous, vulnerable to negative moods, depending on the amount of sugar consumed. Over time, forcing this pattern on the body can result in damaged adrenals.

EMPTY ENERGY

Sugar, in fact, contains virtually no vitamins or minerals. It is empty energy. The body is required to retrieve its B-complex reserves to deal with sugar each time it is ingested. We stress our metabolism by requiring that vitamin sources stored for emergencies (like stress) be retrieved. The continual use of sugar can lead to a vitamin B deficiency. The loss of B[1] (thiamin) interferes with the proper functioning of the nervous system and show up in symptoms of drastic moodiness or constipation. Sugar produces toxic effects and eventually causes cell life to degenerate. It also stimulates an alkali bias in the body which can result in urinary and vaginal infections as well as increase the body's cholesterol count. Thus, while sugar is nutritionally useless, it is not harmless.

....

"I am confident that Western medicine will one day admit what has been known in the Orient for years: sugar is without question the number one murderer in the history of humanity – much more lethal than opium or radioactive fallout. It is the greatest evil that modern industrial civilization has visited upon countries of the Far East and Africa. Foolish people who give or sell candy to babies will one day discover, to their horror, that they have much to answer for."[7]

– Sakurazawa

....

COFFEE AND TEA MAY NOT BE BEST FOR ME

A common series of ingredients consumed by most of the public contain chemicals that, technically speaking, should be classified as drugs. Coffee, tea, cocoa, colas and chocolate contain a powerful and potentially harmful ingredient: caffeine. Caffeine stimulates the metabolism making one feel more awake and active. Depending upon one's susceptibility, however, its ingestion can also produce irregular heartbeats, diarrhea, dwindling concentration, restlessness, increased blood pressure, and other stressful effects. Caffeine inhibits adenosine production in the brain, which then inhibits calmness.

ALL THAT WHITE IS SELDOM NICE

In an attempt to make baked goods that are visually appealing, light, fluffy, and white, grain manufacturers have removed essential nutrients from flour and then bleached the results. Wheat is particularly over-processed. Bleaching agents, preservatives, extenders, and powdered chalk are customarily added to these products. They afford no nutritional value and are indigestible. Hence there is an added stress on the digestive system in attempting to process these foreign items.

For optimum health, try to eat whole grain products as much as possible. Be adventurous; occasionally eat breads made with grains other than wheat.

SALT IN TINY DOSES

Salt is the most favored of spices around the world. It is also one of the most addictive condiments and thus is usually used to excess. Our tongue can get so addictive to excessive salt that without it we feel unable to taste our food.

Salt is a necessary mineral, required for regulating the body's water balance. Sodium aids in the necessary retention of water, yet our body needs extremely small amounts to be healthy. Excessive salt can produce edema, an abnormal accumulation of fluid, which in turn affects blood pressure, driving it up. Salt is very popular in our society; manufacturers routinely add more salt to most prepared food products. Snack foods, of course, are notorious for the large amounts of salt they contain. Chips, pretzels, popcorn, and other salty snack foods are best left for stress diets.

NICOTINE

Although nicotine is not a food, we often associate "a good smoke" with a fine meal, so we'll take a look at it here. While we are all aware of the effects of smoke itself on smokers and bystanders, we may not realize that tobacco also depletes vitamins and distresses the nervous system. In fact, some cigarette manufacturers add sugar to the tobacco and cigarette paper to add 'taste' and ensure that the cigarettes will burn faster. The nervous system is taxed to extreme arousal by nicotine stimulation. In a heavy smoker that arousal state soon becomes the 'normal state'.

Fasting is a wonderful tool to improve your health. It is an ancient form of hygiene, practiced in many cultures. Two things occur during a fast: the body rests from the work of digestion, and the body cleanses itself.

Fasting temporarily stops the accumulation of food to be digested, thus giving the body a chance to "catch up" with its processes of cleansing and reorganize its energy. While digestion rests, elimination is promoted. Toxins and non-nutrients are rounded up from the muscles and fat and eliminated from the body. The bowels empty more thoroughly than usual and vital body functions are stabilized once again. Since all this cleansing is occurring in the body, the mind naturally undergoes a change. It becomes more alert, aware, and uplifted.

Fasting, however, does not mean living on water. It means eliminating all solid food while supplying the body with special liquids to augment its cleansing work. Cleansing juices – made from fresh lemons, oranges, grapefruits, cucumbers and cranberries – flush out the digestive system and remove impurities from the blood and kidneys. Nourishing juices – carrot, apple, lettuce, beet, and other vegetables – provide vitamins, minerals and other nutrients to the body to carry on its work without causing the digestive system to work hard. The use of juices also keeps you from becoming obsessed with the thought of food during the fast.

Traditionally, fasting is done during the change of seasons, especially in the spring and autumn. A three-day fast is then advised. Once a month, or even once a week, a one-day fast can be very beneficial. One can also fast on juices whenever your food or drug consumption, or your mental state has produced sluggishness or excessive toxins.

Fresh fruits and vegetables, organic if possible, should be used to make juices. Non-organic foods should be peeled to remove as much pesticide as possible. The cleansing juices should not be mixed with nourishing juices nor taken right after the other. Cleansing juices should be guzzled to flush out the kidneys. Vegetable juices should be sipped slowly. Cleansing juices for the morning and nourishing juices for the rest of the day should be taken as often as desired.

The transition back to a normal diet after a fast is crucial. Care on the first day is especially important to ensure that the digestive system is gradually re-introduced to solid food. Vegetable broth, plain rice, yogurt, or small amounts of steamed vegetables may be eaten. After a three-to-five day fast, at least two days of these light foods are needed before returning fully to solid foods. Eat small amounts, chew much more than you think necessary, and drink plenty of water.

STRESSLESS EATING

Here are some guidelines to help you establish healthful nutritional habits for optimum wellness:

- **BUY ONLY THE BEST FOOD.**
  Choose food that is as close to its fresh, natural state as possible. The less a food is processed, the more nutrition it retains. Food loses its energy standing on a shelf. Experience this for yourself: cook a can of corn and steam an ear of freshly-picked corn. Eat a few mouthfuls of each. Your taste will discern a radical difference. If you are serious about optimum wellness, choose whole, unprocessed, unpreserved, uncanned foods and demand them from your supermarket.

- **FIND SUGAR SUBSTITUTES.**
  If refined sugar is your addiction become innovative. Substitute natural forms of sweetness like fresh fruit, dried fruit, raisins, even raw carrots. Maple syrup and honey can be eaten in small amounts if you remember that much commercially-prepared honey is made toxic by the processing procedures. Stevia can be selected, a high-powered sweetener without calories. Saccharin and artificial sweeteners belong with the other chemicals: in the garbage.

- **EASY ON DIARY PRODUCTS.**
  If your taste preferences include diary foods, use skimmed. Research would indicate that soy or rice milk is healthier for the body than cow's milk. Remember that cottage cheese, like yogurt, has virtually no fat. Butter is better for your body than the chemicals of margarine. Try cooking with small amounts of clarified butter or extra virgin olive oil.

NEED TO REDUCE?

Crash dieting is quite brutal on the body and emotions. An easier and more effective way to lose weight is through a personal program of exercise and animal fat decrease. Exercise vigorously half an hour at least three or four times per week. This change will improve your overall metabolism and aid your digestive capacities. Eliminate sugar. Drastically minimize fats; bacon and brats do not help the body. If you need a snack, let fruits appease your hunger.

WATCH YOUR PROTEIN.

Books on dieting tend to separate food too rigidly into categories of protein, carbohydrates, fats, etc., implying that each category exists in its pure state in food. Nearly all foods hold mixtures from the other categories. Even lemon juice has protein. Careful with protein: it can imbalance calcium and produce excessive uric acid, inviting a host of intestinal problems. In terms of nutrition, meat is the least important item in your diet. As you get older, consider eliminating red meat and pork entirely, and select from fish, fowl, and vegetable protein. Your digestive tract will last longer.

BECOME MORE SELECTIVE AND VERSATILE.

To insure that you get sufficient vitamins and minerals, compose your menu from a wide variety of vegetables, grains, dried peas and beans, cereals, fruits, fish and lean meat. This abundance and variety was unimaginable thirty years ago, so enjoy more than your mother served.

DO NOT IGNORE WATER.

Fluids constitute most of your body. Fresh, unpolluted water – not canned drinks, tea, or coffee – is welcomed by the kidneys in cleaning the body and aiding the normal body processes. Drink enough water each day so that your urine runs clear at least once a day. Bowel movements can also be improved by drinking sufficient water. Drinking during a meal, however, does not aid digestion but merely dilutes digestive fluids. Wait until you are finished with the meal for your beverage. Gulping ice cold drinks into your hot stomach may relieve your thirst but it strains your digestive and nervous systems.

🍃 BECOME INQUISITIVE.

Food makes your body. So there is no substitute for fresh, unrefined food. Actually, wholesome, well prepared food tends to satisfy the appetite for longer periods than the canned, packaged varieties refined with all sorts of additives. The longer food remains in containers the less vitality it holds for you. The same goes for cooked food that you store. The nutrients diminish while the bulk lingers on. The nutritional destiny of your body is directly proportional to the vitality of your food choices. Read labels.

🍃 ACKNOWLEDGE THE WEATHER.

A cold breakfast is fine in summer but not in winter. During damp, wintry days cold foods stress digestion and put a strain on your body. Let your first meal be warm. Eat more fruit in the summer to cool your body. Anytime you need to be critical and alert, avoid large meals of fried or roasted foods, especially meat.

🍃 INSIDER'S SECRETS.

For longevity and high energy, the advantage goes to those who eat less and drink more water than the norm.

Those in the know do not eat after the sun goes down.

If you are emotionally upset or under pressure, do not eat until you calm down and feel hungry again.

If a food upsets you, refrain no matter how nutritious it is.

Chewing more makes more energy available.

Abundant fresh vegetables and fruits gives you the edge.

🍃 YOUR BODY IS UNIQUE.

Last, and most important, is the indisputable fact that your body is yours. Its uniqueness means that it has certain requirements and tastes that do not correspond to any author's ideal diet. You need to experiment with selections and amounts of foods. Your metabolism is personalized – adjustable, of course, but highly individualized. You may have a stomach that cannot handle mixtures of starches and proteins, so try eating them at separate meals. Your body may not digest fruits eaten with vegetables, so separate their consumption. Your body might be better off with four or five small meals daily rather then the conventional three; you might thrive on just two meals a day.

Breakfast is not the most important meal of the day for everyone unless you like to believe everything the cereal companies (and your mom) propagate. Your nutritional needs have a certain universality about them, but the forms and combinations of food from which you supply these needs is entirely yours to figure out. And they will change as the years move on.

As you begin to pay attention to your food choices, two constant facts will become evident. *First, the quality of the food you ingest profoundly affects the efficiency of your immune system.* A bright, sixteen-year-old girl was brought to see me by her mother. She had begun to fall asleep during high school classes. Her listlessness, as well as many colds, pervaded her semester. An examination of her customary diet exposed the typical fast fried foods (hamburgers and fried bacon), candy, colas, mild shakes, bakery goods, and snacks.

Her face almost went white when I challenged her to an experiment: abandon all of the above for 10 days and instead eat only whole grains, tofu, brown rice, fruits, beans, vegetables, granola, soy patties, and drink loads of water.

Three days later she called me, shocked. Already all her energy and more returned to her with an additional clarity of mind. The enthusiasm grew so much that eventually her grades shot up and she even lost her acne.

The second evident fact is that your body is mostly water. We forget the need to drink plenty of water to our peril as we grow older. The best thing we can do for our health is to gradually increase our pure water consumption, to two or more quarts a day. Research indicates that chronic dehydration, like high blood pressure, sabotages wellness more then one can suspect and is a hidden precursor to diseases. In a fascinating book, *Your Body's Many Cries For Water*, Dr. Batmanghelidj[8] narrates how he was utterly surprised by curing 3000 peptic ulcer patients and other degenerative diseases by simply upgrading their intake of water with a small amount of salt.

Over lunch one day, my Aikido partner and long-time friend, Maynard, was curious about what constituted a wellness diet. Could someone afford it without being a millionaire? I suggested that we take an educational walk through Kowalski's Market. So after lunch we went shopping.

On Maynard's suggested budget of $50.00 for a week of food, we bought the following: broccoli, tomatoes, onions, mushrooms, potatoes, yams, garlic, green peppers, celery, spinach, lettuce, sweet corn, carrots, cherries, peaches, apricots, bananas, plums, cantaloupe, strawberries, soy milk, butter, cheese, eggs, vermicelli noodles, okara patties, tofu, olive oil, Italian sauce, rice, dry beans, oatmeal, bread, crackers, and frozen fruit juice. The bill amounted to $50.11.

We then discussed that a typical week with our groceries could produce breakfasts of cereal, fruit, eggs, or toast; main meals of spaghetti and salad, tofu with vegetables, rice and beans with vegetables, okra patties and vegetables; small meals of salad, bread, cheese sandwiches, soup made from the extra vegetables, and fruit for dessert. Water and fruit juice could be drunk throughout the day.

Next week one could purchase nuts, dried fruit, different dried lentils, and a treat of fruit sorbet or healthy cookies, since some of the staples would last longer than a week. Instead of oatmeal, for instance, one could make granola.

I handed the two shopping bags of groceries to my incredulous friend who was mumbling, "I didn't think it was possible," and sent him home to begin.

PRACTICE SESSION

Food Diary

Strange as it may seem, many people are unaware of the composition of their diet on a day-to-day basis. Most sense whether the meals are tasty or not, but make no discernment or reflection on their contents.

For your own information and guidance in food wellness, keep a notebook with you all the time and jot down everything you put in your mouth for a week. Write down the time of eating, the name of the food, and the amount consumed. Note sizes of portions, helpings, or snacks. Do the same with everything you drink. After listing what you ate, list how you feel during the ensuing minutes.

After a week, review your approach to nutrition. Read your entire list and note any patterns. What times of the day do you eat? Do you eat on impulse? Are certain foods irresistible? What snacks? Note especially how you felt during the hour following ingestion. Were you more alert? Sluggish? Feeling heavy? In other words, what mood resulted from eating?

When you reflect on the week's diary, note if there are motivation patterns forming. Do you eat sometimes out of boredom? Stress? Loneliness? Do you use alcohol to get rid of tensions? Are you stuck on coffee? How do you approach food during a hectic day? Could you face the day without stimulants? Are you terribly upset if you miss a meal? Do you feel sleepy or irritable after eating certain foods?

The whole point of the diary is not to incriminate yourself but to become a resource for self-knowledge. The quality of energy you eat and drink shows up in your body and in its feelings. The nutrition you assimilate makes you feel certain ways about yourself. Armed with the experiential knowledge of your personal choices in nutrition, you will have more freedom to make the necessary changes towards your wellness in your diet.

CHAPTER 5

Movement:
Action for Awareness

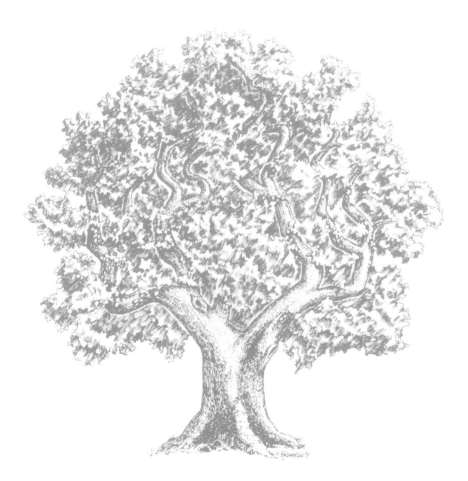

As we have seen, your physical body is structured energy. Every portion of that energy contains information that feeds back to your mind: you can sense the temperature of your skin, you can feel the tension of muscles as you chew food, walk up stairs, lift a heavy parcel, or scratch your neck. You can sense when you have extra energy and when you over-extend your endurance. Whatever physical activities you do, your body communicates its energy status to your mind. Just learn to pay attention

Since your body is an extension of your mind, both work in very close conjunction. What one does immediately affects the other. Your body is always aware of subtle signals from your mind, and your mind is always aware of changes in your body, even when your conscious, rational mind is not aware of them. Your unconscious mind is always sending and receiving signals to and from the energy you call your body and sending it to your conscious mind. If, however, you habitually over-stress the body, accumulating patterns of emotional and muscular tension, you can eventually reach a stage where you constrain the marvelous sensitivity of the body/mind communication.

That loss of sensitivity is, in a way, a compensation for the condition of stress. In that state you would not think you were exhausted, or stressed, or nervous because you would no longer feel the signals of stress. You could even adjust to this diminished condition of energy, accepting it as your norm. Then you might walk around in tension, not realizing your body/mind distress until it became extreme and you were forced to take notice, when stiffness or a serious illness stopped you in your tracks.

If you want to have optimum wellness, the inter-communication between your body and mind must be improved and strengthened.

How can you strengthen your mind's perception of the energy status of your body? How can your mind make better use of that energy? How does the body improve its performance of the mind's directions? It is accomplished through reflective exercise.

WHY EXERCISE?

Exercise can reorganize the energy of your body and mind. It can rechannel fatigue to useful energy. At first glance, this assertion seems illogical. When your muscles feel tense from the stress of the day, or your mind is weary from various problems, it seems highly unlikely that vigorous movement would reduce the tension. While it is true that someone in an exhaustive condition needs rest, everyday tiredness responds very positively to action. Moderate exercise erodes the accumulated patterns of stress by reconstituting its energy.

When you use your muscles vigorously, the embedded sedentary and stressed patterns loosen their restrictions in your body. Vigorous exercise can heighten the communication between mind and body and recharges the body. Changing the routine of your body changes your routine of awareness. Pay attention. A brisk walk, jogging, a few laps around the pool, can all rid the body of toxins and reawaken your energy. Exercising over a period of time makes your body begin to feel better, and helps your mind to feel relaxed and enthusiastic. Your mental energy improves by inducing graceful and strong movements. This improvement in body/mind communication wards off the chronic buildup of stress. When your body is energized through movement, it increases its efficiency as a living instrument. Not only do you function better physically and emotionally, but your recovery time from exertion is shortened.

....

Studies show that the combination of aerobic exercise plus resistance training accelerates the loss of fat without loss of necessary muscle. "A toned muscle can gobble calories like a piranha fish ... muscle is still working when at rest, and its caloric-burning can leap as much as 20-fold when put into action."[1]

....

With its system of over 600 muscles, your body is designed for action. Muscles thrive on being used. Unless there is severe atrophy or paralysis, improvement in muscle tone and suppleness is possible at any age. An injured muscle heals even faster when it is carefully used than when it is inactive. We know that recovery from heart problems proceeds better with intelligent exercise than with inactivity, chiefly because the heart is a muscle. We can extend this principle of healing through activity to the entire body by stating that health and well-being are enhanced by sufficient, regular exercise.

A New England medical study focused on a group of rather frail nursing home residents, aged 86 to 96. The subjects were taught to use weight resistance machines and their strength was then measured. Three times a week the ten men and women exercised with 24 leg lifts. They started at 50% of their maximum load and after a week advanced to 80%. After two months, all the participants measured a three- to four-fold increase in leg strength. Two subjects also were able to walk easily without their canes, one regained the strength to rise without assistance, and four increased their walking speed by 48%.[2]

From the perspective of stress and wellness, there are four major benefits produced by an intelligent program of exercise:

MOVEMENT DETOXES THE BODY.
By embarking on a daily or frequent regime of exercise – one that leads to perspiration – your entire metabolism improves. Your skin is the largest organ in your body and sweating is one of the methods your body uses to rid itself of various toxins that deplete energy. The vigorous breathing used during exercise also helps the immune system to ward off disease by stimulating the lymphatic process, thus cleaning the toxins from the body.

RHYTHMIC MOVEMENT OVERCOMES FATIGUE.
Our bodies love rhythm. The heart beats in rhythm, the lungs inflate and deflate in rhythm, the organs secrete and move in a regular beat. Thus, it is no surprise that sustained motion with a sense of rhythm and fun is the chief tool for dispersing fatigue. Generating energy through exercise replaces tiredness with stimulation of organs and

nerves. Vigorous motion reorganizes the flow of your energy and tones your heart, lungs, and limbs, along with your circulatory and digestive systems. In fact, it has been discovered that with proper diet, rest and regular exercise, your heart can even grow its own bypass channels when other arteries remain blocked.

If you are afflicted with chronic fatigue, however, where weariness pervades your days, then exercise is not your prescription. For you, restoration through rest is the priority. Follow the practices in the chapter on rest and come back to movement when your body has caught up a bit.

✐ MOVEMENT IMPROVES MOOD.

Your mood can be drastically influenced by exercise. Since movement alters the flow of energy through your entire body, it lifts you from a sense of emotional weariness to one of emotional well-being. Once you get used to doing regular exercise the memory of how you feel during and afterwards becomes an incentive to continue exercising. Even brief exercise counterbalances moodiness and depression fades with sustained exercise. The activated energy patterns of physical pleasure lay the foundation for the changeover.

✐ MOVEMENT INDUCES RELAXATION OF BODY AND MIND.

Research shows that the degree of relaxation improves when one first tenses the body and then releases that tension, rather than directly attempting to relax. Drs. P. Insel and W. Roth of Stanford University say that, "the most profound muscular and mental relaxation cannot be achieved by just trying to relax. The deepest relaxation, as measured by electrodes inserted in the muscles, follows a period of voluntarily increased muscle tension."[3]

The key here is that the entire process must be done with voluntary attention. Relaxation is best done systematically throughout the body to insure that the major regions of the body are benefited and none are forgotten. Exercise, particularly stretching exercises which involve contraction and release, insures this cycle.

Inactivity is very stressful for your body and mind; ennui produces much more stress than exercise. After strenuous, but not exhausting, aerobic movement, you will feel a sense of pleasant tiredness and calm vigor.

During the day you put your body and its sensory-motor systems through many stresses and strains. Your body responds with specific muscular reflexes. Over time these repeated reflexes become habitual muscular contractions which interfere with your relaxation. The muscular contractions then become customary to our posture, a kind of signature whereby our friends recognize us as we sit, stand, and walk. The only trouble with this process is that our posture and movement produces joint stiffness and muscle soreness. We forget how to move freely. We have become candidates for somatic amnesia: the inability to remember the potentials of the body. We now think the decrements of aging – loss of flexibility, general aches and pains, a reduction of body/mind communication – are inevitable and natural.

We forget how to move freely.

The path to decrepitude is strewn with slogans: "You're not getting any younger, you know." "All things do break down." "Well, it's normal for my age." "You really ought to slow down." "Don't forget your age, you're not so young anymore." Typically physicians attribute to the notion of "aging" a host of debilitations that seemingly overtake anyone over forty. Physician and patient easily assign these symptoms to "age" as the indomitable, irreversible culprit, setting up a superstitious co-dependency: take your drugs to relieve the pain; its the most you can do.

Surprise! Aging does not automatically deteriorate vitality. Dr. Gavin of Concordia University tells us that even ten minutes of extra activity per day can reduce the risk of heart disease by 50%. According to the summary of a full body of research done on aging and the brain, "… there is no generalization about neuron loss in old age."[4]

We grow weak, passive and decay not because of our age but because we plan the obsolescence of our bodies. Most elder people with impaired motor performance, slowness, loss of strength and coordination have built attrition into their lifestyle. As a general adage, most structural impairments, from low back pain to arthritic joints and restricted mobility, are functional challenges, rather than structural deformities. Maladies of old age are mostly maladaptations: one forfeits the functional use of physical abilities by refusing to stimulate the brain. Damage occurs not through degeneration but through the loss of internal awareness.

Fortunately, the ensemble of symptoms from somatic amnesia are not necessarily permanent. When a physician declares that you have "reduced nerve impulse activity related to progressive disuse together with functional impairment and subsequent loss of motoreurones," he or she is alerting you to "move it or lose it."

Medical treatment does not remedy the dysfunction nor do drugs restore the body/mind communication; re-education does. If your body has been allowed to become dormant, you must increase and reawaken the consciousness of feeling through voluntary movement. Your stiff reflexes and sore muscles are a learned adaptive response which can be reversed. To do this, you must increase voluntary control over your body through movement. Hatha yoga, the Feldenkrais method of movement (based on yoga), and the systematic contraction and release of muscles are excellent ways to rejuvenate your flexibility.

CORPORATE FITNESS AND WELLNESS

Wellness emphasizes optimal living. It places a premium on the individual's natural desire to actualize those potentials of body, emotions, and mind that promote a healthy and active lifestyle. Surprisingly, by introducing wellness programs, businesses are realizing a positive cost-benefit ratio that exceeds expectations. Less absenteeism and employee turnover, reduced training costs, and lower sickness claims are only some of the long term pay back results.

....

"The evidence pointing to the success of fitness programs in improving employee health practices, reducing medical and disability costs, and improving productivity is indisputable."[5]
– Kenneth Pelletier, Ph.D.

....

The following are some advantages noted by corporations when they adopted a corporate wellness and fitness program for their employees:

- OVER A SIX YEAR PERIOD Du Pont reduced absences due to illnesses by 14 per cent and received a return of $2.06 per dollar invested in its program.

- EXERCISERS ARE LESS LIKELY to leave the Tenneco corporation in Houston. The company noted that it attracted more health-conscious employees than other companies. The average annual medical claim for wellness participants is 50 per cent lower than other employees.

- AT&T PROJECTS SAVINGS of 87 million dollars from reduced heart disease and cancers.

- BLUE CROSS AND BLUE SHIELD of Indiana found savings of $519.00 per participant, a benefit to cost ratio of 2.51–1.

- SCOULAR GRAIN CO. in Omaha saved over $1 million in 1989 in health care costs – $1500.00 per employee.

- JOHNSON & JOHNSON saved $378.00 per employee with lower absenteeism.

- CONTROL DATA estimates over 10 years a $4.00 return per every $1.00 invested.

- MOTOROLA returned $3.15 per dollar invested.

- OVER FOUR YEARS Kennecott Copper realized $5.78 per each dollar invested.

- NORTHERN GAS CO. showed that participants had 80 per cent fewer sick days.

- CANADIAN LIFE ASSURANCE noted a 32.4 per cent lower rate of absenteeism over a seven year period compared with non-participants.

- TORONTO LIFE ASSURANCE found during a 10 month period a 15 per cent decline in absenteeism.

- NASA FOUND wellness participants to have improved stamina and work performance along with enhanced concentration and decision abilities. While average efficiency decreases 50 per cent in the last two hours of the working day, exercise participants showed full efficiency, which amounted to a 12.5 per cent increase in productivity.

- AT SAATCHI & SAATCHI 75 per cent of participants affirmed an improved morale. Sixty-three per cent of participants felt more relaxed, patient, and less tired during the day at The Canadian Life Assurance Co.

- AT GENERAL ELECTRIC, employees who exercised were absent from work 45 per cent fewer days than non-exercisers. Dupont, the Dallas Police Department and General Mills had improvements from 14 per cent to 80 per cent.

- A NINE-MONTH Purdue University study of 80 people found that exercisers increased their ability to make complex decisions by 70 per cent.

- IN THE MASTER MILE at the Sunkist Invitational track meet in Los Angeles, 53-year-old Sid Howard ran at 4: 43.7. His best time when in High School was 4:48.[6]

TYPES OF EXERCISE

Exercise can be generally divided into four major categories:

1. ISOTONIC MOVEMENT.
   These are the exercises concerned with building muscle strength by using strenuous load bearing movements. Weight lifting, gymnastics, and rowing are typical forms. Movement of the muscles through space, combining contraction and extension qualifies as isotonic movement. While a routine of isotonic exercises invigorates the muscles, the internal systems still need additional stimulation.

2. ISOMORPHIC MOVEMENT.
   In these exercises the muscles do not get extended as in lifting weights; they are simply contracted and held that way for some seconds before being released. Typical examples would be pushing or pulling against stationary objects, pressing ones' hands together, attempting to lift the chair while sitting on it. A series of simple muscular contractions takes very little time to perform and can be done almost anywhere

   Interestingly, the contraction of a muscle for seven to ten seconds, repeated three times in succession, produces an enormous change in

the energy pattern of the contracted area. Exercise physiologists have recorded a sixty percent increase in muscle strength in less than three months of daily practice with isomorphic movement.

3. AEROBIC MOVEMENT.

Aerobic exercise is that which increases the efficiency of oxygen intake. In practice, this means that you moderate the speed of your movement so that you do not become so out of breath that you must cease the motion. The heart pumps and lungs breathe more intensely but you do not bring yourself to the stage of breathlessness, or what is called oxygen debt. With practice, your bodily stamina improves as the cardio-vascular system becomes strengthened. Some physicians tell us that even a few minutes of extra activity per day can reduce one's risk of heart disease by fifty percent.

During aerobics the entire body is stimulated, particularly the heart and lungs. The oxygen capacity increases and purifies the blood. The heart, lungs, and circulation are toned. More and more energy is available, and the body feels more and more energetic. Typical aerobic movements are jogging, dancing, swimming, hiking, brisk walking, cycling, bouncing, and sets of stair-climbing.

Substantial physical improvements occur when the duration of aerobic movement is sustained for twenty to thirty minutes, at least three times weekly. These short, frequent periods of exercise are more beneficial than a long session once a week. The key to gaining optimum benefit from aerobics is to be playful while exercising. Leave seriousness and harsh competition in your locker.

4. STRETCHING MOVEMENTS.

Stretching keeps the body exceedingly fit by stretching and twisting the muscles, ligaments, sinews and joints while massaging the internal organs. Body flexibility and suppleness are improved and, as a bonus, the internal organs are toned up.

Superior among all stretching movement is hatha yoga. Many illnesses can be prevented or healed by a systematic regimen of hatha yoga. The twisting and bending motion of these exercises is performed slowly and with full attention. No strain is involved and breathing is never accelerated. Maximum benefit ensues when breathing is synchronized with the motion of the body. Balance, coordination, and communication between mind and body is then vastly improved.

BEGINNING A ROUTINE

As we become older, combinations of aerobics, isomorphics, isotonics, and stretching are recommended most particularly for achieving optimum wellness. A sedentary lifestyle tends to stiffen the body, impedes the natural processes of the internal organs and erodes our flexibility, balance, and resistance to stress. Obviously, when our bodies are fit we are unlikely to succumb to sudden physical stresses and strains that seem to plague older adults. It is up to us to claim that fitness through movement.

Initiate your exercise program carefully. If you have not been exercising vigorously for some time, begin with light-heartedness and pace yourself as you go by how you feel. The workout should leave you with a good feeling of tiredness but not fatigue. At first you will experience some soreness or stiffness. That's where the stretching comes in. Gentle stretches before and after your aerobics will alleviate the pain. Remember that extreme intensity may make you feel like you have accomplished a goal, but excessive pain leads to injury, loss of interest, and useless stress. Grimness produces strain and removes enjoyment from your workout. Take your time in warming into the motions and easing off at their completion. Tailor your activity in reference to your age and circumstances.

One of the most important aspects for your personal exercise program is the issue of goal. You must decide your objective: Do you want fitness? If so, take the long-range approach. Be playful and patient. Do you want competitive conditioning? If so, then you will have to mix a lot of anaerobic (you should get out of breath) movements into your workout.

Experiment with your body to find out which exercises make you feel the pleasure of physical vigor. You need to find out what suits your taste in movement, goals, and outside weather conditions. When becoming fit appears a chore, make it playful. If there are many demands on your energy, you may tend to forego the regular activity of exercise when pressed for time. And because you feel tired from the day, you might not think that exercise is appropriate for reviving your energy. Only by experimenting can you discover whether or not exercise in the face of general tiredness can revitalize your energy. Fitness, by and large, is a matter of regularity and appropriate intensity. Finally, be aware of how you are treating yourself by this activity. Are you exercising to augment your health or are you creating another variation of stress? Think twice about getting involved with competing against the clock, against your partner or against an ideal number of repetitions. Like your other resource tools, keep exercise in context: fitness is not an end in itself, but an enjoyable and healthful portion of life. Let it assist you by supplying the energy for your larger goals.

PRACTICE SESSION

Yoga Postures

The following practice is a sequence of joints and glands exercises and hatha yoga postures. They should be practiced in the order listed so that major body parts are prepared for the more difficult postures, and all areas of the body are included. Do not get out of breath nor allow yourself to feel any mounting sense of strain. Start each practice recognizing your current degree of flexibility and move with it. Rest between postures to return your breath to normal. The postures should be performed very slowly and carefully, with full attention. Always stretch only until you reach your capacity so that you do not strain yourself. Your body will let you know when you can go a little further. End the practice session with a full relaxation in the corpse posture.

NOTE: The postures are available on cassette tape. See order page.

NECK BENDS

Stand or sit erect. While exhaling, slowly drop your head to your chest. Do not move your shoulders. Inhaling, slowly raise your head and drop it backwards, pointing your chin towards the ceiling. Exhale and return to center.

Exhale slowly and turn your head as far as possible to the right. Try to bring your chin over your shoulder, but do not move your shoulders. Inhale slowly and return to center.

Exhale and turn your head as far as possible to the left, bringing your chin over your left shoulder. Inhale and return to center.

Exhale and slowly lower your head to the right, trying to bring your ear to your right shoulder without raising your shoulder. Inhale and return to center.

Exhale while lowering your head to the left, and try to bring your left ear to your left shoulder without raising your shoulder. Inhale and return to center.

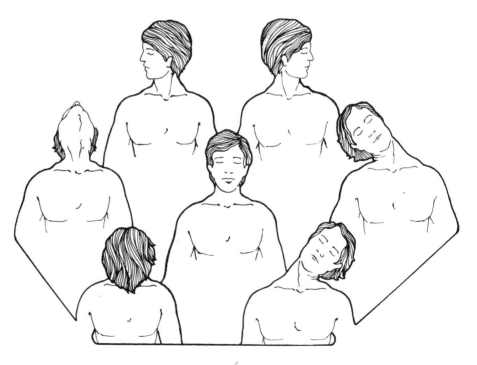

ARM SWINGS

Stand erect. Raise your arms out to your sides at shoulder level. With an exhalation, swing your arms forward, crossing the right over the left. Pull your shoulders together to separate your shoulder blades. With an inhalation, swing your arms out past the sides to the back, crossing the right over the left. Pull shoulders together to expand your chest.

Repeat three times with your right arm over the left and three times with your left arm over the right.

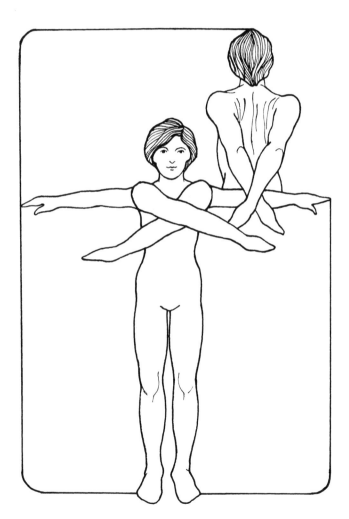

WALL PUSH UPS

Stand erect facing a wall, about one foot away from it. Place your hands on the wall at shoulder level. Slowly walk backwards until your body is at a 45 degree angle. Keep your legs straight. Bend your arms at the elbow, leaning into the wall and stretching the calf muscles. Breathe evenly for three breaths.

Extend your arms and repeat the exercise.

Next, bend your arms, leaning into the wall, but this time bend your knees forward, stretching the lower Achilles' tendon. Hold for three breaths. Return to the first position and repeat again.

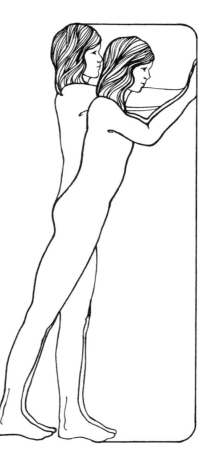

OVERHEAD STRETCH

Stand erect, arms at sides. With an inhalation, raise your arms up over your head. Keep your palms together and your ears between your upper arms.

Without lifting your heels off the floor, stretch up from your legs, pelvis, chest and arms as high as you can, as if you were reaching for the ceiling with your fingertips.

With an exhalation, lower your arms and relax your body.

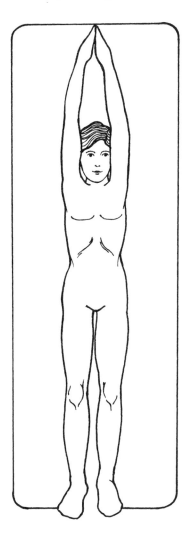

KNEE SWIRL

Stand erect with your hands on your hips.

Raise your right leg until your thigh is parallel to the floor. Relax your leg, letting all the muscles below the knee hang loosely. Swing your leg below the knee in a clockwise direction, keeping the thigh still.

Repeat in a counterclockwise direction.

Lower the leg to the floor and repeat the swirls with your left leg.

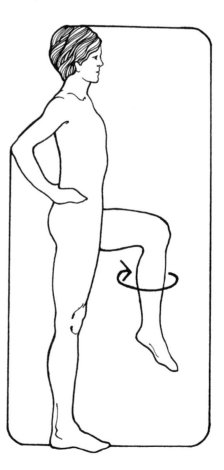

ANKLE ROLLS

Stand erect with your hands on your hips.

Shift your body weight to the left leg. Keeping the right leg straight, raise it a few inches off the floor. Bending your right foot at the ankle, move it to point the toes up towards the ceiling, then down towards the floor.

Still standing on your left foot, move your right foot to point the toes to the right as far as possible and then to the left.

Next, slowly rotate the right foot at the ankle in a clockwise direction and then in a counterclockwise direction.

Finally, lower your right foot to the floor and relax the muscles.

Repeat the entire exercise with your left foot.

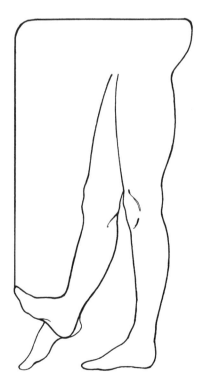

DANCING KNEES

Stand erect, hands on your hips, feet about ten inches apart.

By tensing the muscles above and surrounding your right knee cap, raise your knee cap.

Relax the muscles and let the knee cap return to its normal position.

Repeat with the left knee cap. Begin slowly and increase the speed of the motion until the kneecaps appear to dance up and down. Continue to 'dance' the knees for about one minute.

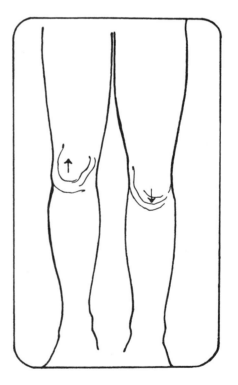

LEG KICKS

Stand erect, hands on hips.

Shift your body weight to your left leg and raise your right leg slightly off the floor. Point your toes forward and with a quick movement, swing your right leg back to kick your buttocks.

Relax the leg, bringing it down close to the floor, and then repeat the kick again up to about ten times.

Lower your right foot, shift body weight to your right leg and kick ten times with your left leg.

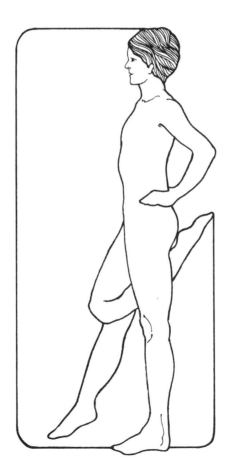

POSTERIOR STRETCH

Sit erect with your legs extended together in front of your body. With an inhalation, raise your arms overhead.

With an exhalation, stretch up and bend forward, keeping your back straight and your head between your arms. Grasp your big toes and bring your head toward your shins, elbows on the floor alongside the knees.

Breathe evenly for three breaths.

With the next inhalation, slowly return to a sitting position.

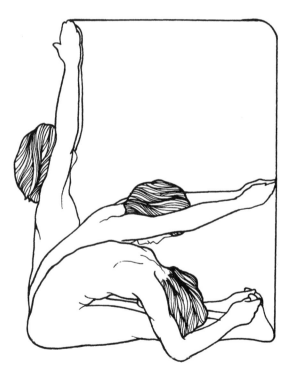

THE WELLNESS TREE

SPREAD LEGS

Sit erect with your legs spread as far apart as possible, hands resting on your knees.

With an inhalation, raise your arms out to the sides at shoulder level. With an exhalation, bend forward from the hips, trying to rest your chin on the floor. Grasp the instep of each foot.

Breathe evenly for two to three breaths. With an inhalation, slowly return to a sitting position. Be sure to keep your spine straight and flat during this posture.

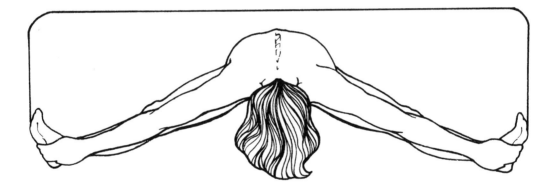

COBRA

Lie face downward with your forehead touching the floor, legs together. Place your hands, palms down, close to your body, fingers aligned with your nipples.

With an inhalation, slowly raise your head, brushing first your nose, then your chin against the floor. Continue the motion, lifting your neck, shoulders, and chest. Look up and back as far as possible.

Breathe evenly for three breaths. Your thorax should be lifted by the back muscles only and not by pushing with the arms. Your body from the navel down should be flat on the floor and relaxed.

With an exhalation, slowly lower your body, chest first, then shoulders, neck, and head, until your forehead is resting on the floor.

Relax and repeat.

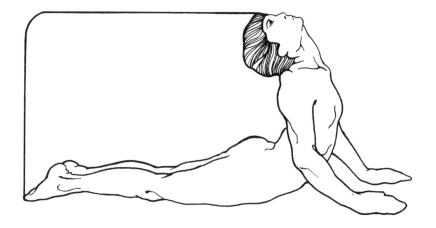

CHILD'S POSE

Sit in a kneeling position with the top of your feet on the floor and your buttocks resting on your heels. Keep your head, neck, and trunk in a straight line. Relax your arms and rest your hands on the floor, palms upward, fingers pointing behind you.

Exhaling, bend forward from the hips until your abdomen and chest are resting on your thighs and your forehead touches the floor in front of you. Slide the hands and arms back into a comfortable position, close to the body.

Relax fully and breathe deeply.

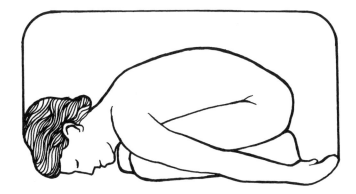

TRIANGLE

Stand erect, arms at sides, legs three feet apart. With an inhalation, raise your arms to shoulder level, palms down, and twist your torso to the right.

With an exhalation, bend forward, placing your left hand alongside the right foot and extend the right arm straight up. Move your chin over the right shoulder and look up at the right hand. Be sure not to bend the knees. Breathe evenly for three breaths. With an inhalation, slowly raise to the standing position, arms at shoulder level.

Return to center and catch your breath. Repeat the bend on the left side, bringing the right hand alongside your left foot.

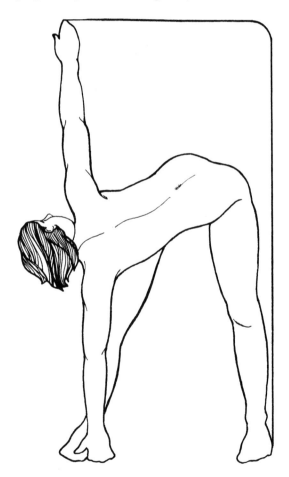

KING DANCER

Stand erect, arms at sides and legs together. With an exhalation, bend your left leg and grasp the instep with the left hand, pulling your foot close to your buttocks. Inhale and lift your right arm straight up.

With an exhalation, tilt your torso, head, and right arm forward as a unit. With the next inhalation, pull up the shoulder blades together while holding the posture for three breaths. With the next exhalation, slowly lower your right arm, release your left ankle, and repeat the posture on the other side.

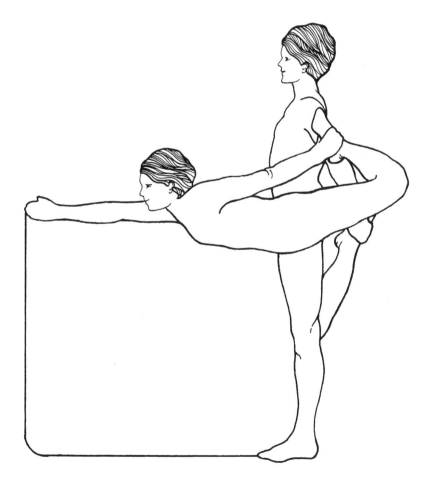

MONKEY

Stand erect, hands at sides. Extend your left leg behind your body, bending at the right knee. Lower your body until the left foot, shin, and knee are flat on the floor and your right leg is perpendicular to the floor.

With an inhalation, raise your arms overhead, palms together. With an exhalation, gently bend back and look up at your hands. Breathe evenly for three breaths. Slowly return to the standing position and repeat the posture on the other side.

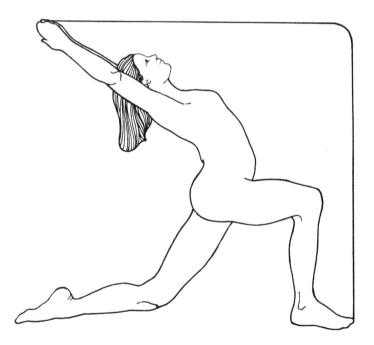

HALF SPINAL TWIST

Sit erect with your legs extended in front of your body. Bend your right leg and place the heel of your right foot against your perineum, the area between the anus and the genitals.

Bend the left leg, move your left foot over your right knee and place it on the floor on the outside of the right knee. With an inhalation, lift your arms to shoulder level.

With an exhalation, twist your body to the left, past the upright left knee, and grasp your left foot with your right hand. Wrap your left arm around your back to grasp your waist. Move your chin over your left shoulder.

Breathe evenly for three breaths. Return to the original position and repeat the posture on the other side.

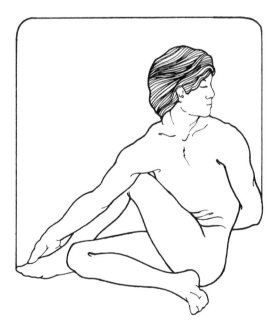

TWISTING POSTURE

Lie on your back, legs together, arms stretched out, palms down at shoulder level. With an inhalation, bend your knees and bring your legs up to your chest.

With an exhalation, slowly lower your bent legs to the floor at your right elbow, while turning your head as far as possible to the left. Shoulders should remain on the floor. Breathe evenly for three breaths.

With an inhalation, return your knees and head to the center. With the next exhalation, lower your bent legs to the floor at your left elbow, while turning your head as far as possible to the right.

Repeat the exercise three times.

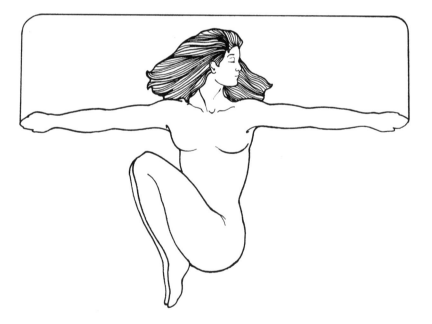

LEG LIFTS

Lie on your back, legs together, hands at your sides, palms down. With an inhalation, raise your right leg as high as possible. Do not bend your knees.

Hold for three breaths. With an exhalation, slowly lower your leg.

With an inhalation, raise your left leg as high as possible.

Hold for three breaths. With an exhalation, slowly lower your leg.

With another inhalation, raise both legs, keeping them straight.

Hold for three breaths. With an exhalation, slowly lower both legs. Repeat.

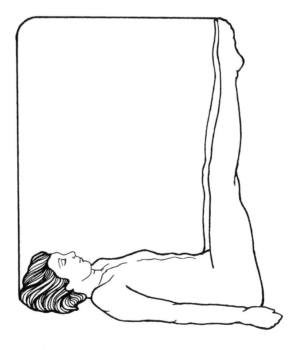

SHOULDER STAND

Lie on your back, arms to the sides and legs together.

With an inhalation, slowly raise your legs perpendicular to the floor. Then lift your trunk to a vertical position while raising your hands and forearms to support your back. Your chin should press against the breastbone; your legs should be together; the entire body should be in a straight line.

Breathe evenly for three breaths.

With an exhalation, slowly come out of the posture by gently lowering your legs slightly over your head, replacing your forearms and hands on the floor and lowering your trunk and legs.

Relax. Increase the time in this posture until you can hold it comfortably for one minute.

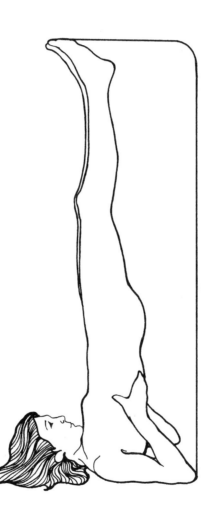

PLOW

Lie on your back, arms at your sides and legs together. With an inhalation, slowly raise your legs perpendicular to the floor without bending your knees. Press your palms against the floor. Bring your legs back, raising your hips and then your back off the floor.

Keeping your legs together, slowly lower them toward the floor behind your head. Your arms remain on the floor.

Breathe evenly for three breaths while holding this posture.

With an exhalation, slowly lower your back, hips, and legs to the floor. Relax.

Increase the time in this posture until you can hold it comfortably for one minute.

Be careful not to overextend in this pose.

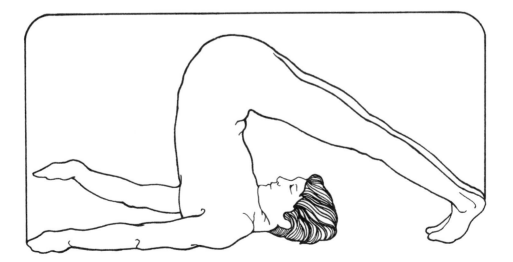

THE BRIDGE

Lie on your back, arms at your sides, palms down, legs together. Bend at the knees and slide your feet toward your body until your heels touch your buttocks.

With an inhalation, raise your hips and torso off the floor as high as possible. Feet, hands, shoulders, and head remain on the floor.

Breathe evenly for three breaths.

With an exhalation, slowly lower your hips and torso to the floor. Relax.

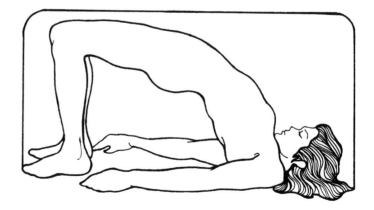

THE HALF FISH

Lie on the floor with your feet together, arms by your sides and your head in a straight line with your body.

With an inhalation, slowly expand and lift your chest off the floor by arching your back. Slide your arms up until your elbows and palms are resting on the floor at your sides. Stretch your neck open in front and rest the crown of your head on the floor.

Breathe evenly for three to six breaths.

Slowly remove the pressure from your elbows by straightening your back, releasing your neck and head, and lying full on the floor.

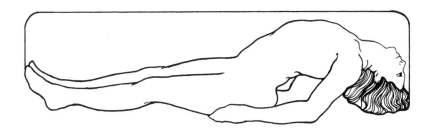

KNEES TO CHEST

Lie on your back, legs extended.

Bend your legs and bring them to your chest. Wrap your arms around your legs, pulling them as close as possible to your chest. If there is any pain in your lower back, rock gently from side to side.

Next, extend your right leg to the floor, hold the left leg to your chest, and bring your forehead to the knee.

Breathe evenly for three breaths.

Return to the prone position and repeat with your other leg.

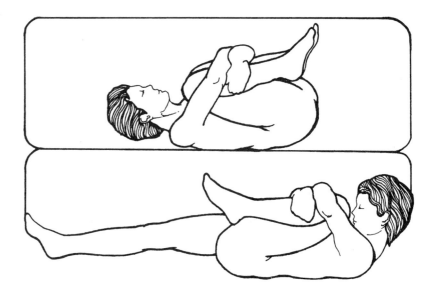

CORPSE POSE

Lie on your back, legs about two feet apart, arms about eight inches from your body, palms up. Your head, neck, and trunk should be in a straight line.

Close your eyes and relax your body completely.

Breathe evenly and deeply for three to five minutes.

This posture should always complete any exercise series and is also the posture for several relaxation exercises.

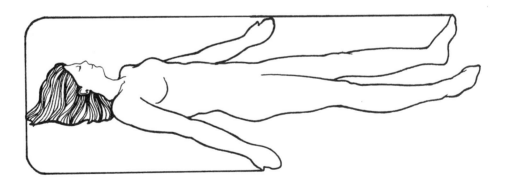

CHAPTER 6

Rest:
Don't Decline to Recline

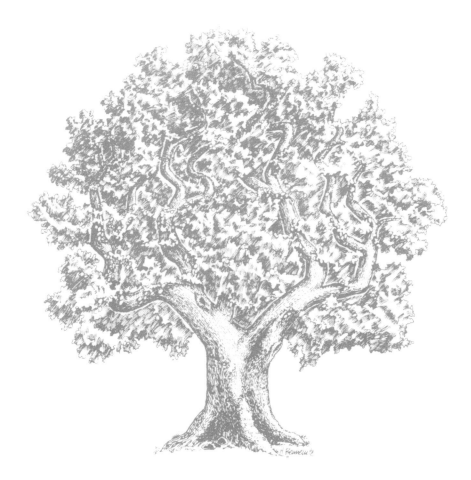

Some centuries ago, a famous Greek philosopher remarked that the most obvious fact about life is that it changes. Upon this undeniable fact he composed one of the first scientific treatises on the nature of change. Brilliant as he was, Aristotle never imagined the pace of cultural changes you and I encounter in our lives: the 24-hour, last-minute-rush kind of changes. Our lives are changing much faster today than those of any of our ancestors.

The challenge of change is a stranger to no one. We all experience change in at least some of its manifold forms. In fact, without change we would die. Our cell life is limited to only a few weeks of existence.

Life and change go hand in hand. The more we contact life, the more we are introduced to change on a grand, never-ending scale. Life's slightest touch can alter our thoughts and feelings. Those changes provoke emotions. Whether we like, approve, and accept a change or dislike, disapprove, and resist the same change, we generate emotion.

Our language indicates this emotional contact. We say we are "moved" or "touched" by an incident. The Greeks called that feeling the "suffering of life." By suffering they do not necessarily mean distress, but emotional change. When you contact life's events, the energy of your emotions fluctuates, and you move from one emotional condition to a new one. Whether you enjoy a positive experience like laughter, or resent a negative experience like frustration, the result is the same: an energy transition occurs. You feel the difference and you feel differently about yourself. As the Greeks say, you have "suffered."

Change often provokes stress. A mother suffers childbirth with mixed emotions. Her acute pain and her joyful relief are inseparable.

They compose her memorable, emotional, and stressful experience. At her child's birth, her months-long distress recedes into the joy of the new life. Her body heals itself while retaining the memory of the pain.

Five years later the woman celebrates her child's birthday with all the neighborhood kids. The party produces excitement in the children and smiling pride in the parents. But everyone at the party experiences their emotions. Sooner or later the enjoyment wearies because prolonged or quick emotional change can tire the body. With energy flagging, stress soon abounds. The kids become whiny and complaining, the parents stop smiling. Stress ends the event.

Of course none of us would want to avoid stressful experiences by denying the fun of life, but it is helpful to recognize that either change for the better or change for the worse occasions emotional stress. Living high, or living low, being in charge or being driven, having a good time or feeling miserable, all accumulate their toll.

Then how should we balance stress and activity? How do we help accumulated stress to diminish?

COPING WITH EMPTY ENERGY

Typically, busy people complain about stress in their lives but shy away from its resolution. The average busy person begs: "What can I do? I don't have time for rest." Neither did Mrs. Grindhorse.

After three appointments with two physicians, Mrs. Grindhorse walked into my London office. A pleasant, smartly dressed woman of forty-two, she had started a new window accessory business five years earlier with her husband. The business expanded faster than anticipated and she hired additional help. Her husband noted how competent and devoted she was to business cares and 'graciously handed more and more of his duties to her while he went off to the pub or the local fishing spot. Her daughter, who worked in the business only infrequently, was currently involved with the latest drug fad and preferred to stay stoned. Her gentle Asian employees had the habit of failing to show up for work whenever they celebrated their many cultural holidays. Being very conscientious, Mrs. Grindhorse absorbed the employee slack by taking their duties on herself and putting in hours and hours of overtime. Soon, besides being the working chairwoman and proprietor, she was manager, saleswoman, buyer, accountant, and janitor. Although she resented the extra work, she was too kind to complain to her family, even while she continued to be responsible for the lion's share of the household duties. It was unfair but what could she do? She kept all her emotions inside her. Sleep became fitful as she rehearsed the business agenda. Fatigue and vague distress became constant companions. She began to experience chest pains.

Physicians could not find any functional impairment, so they recommended mild tranquilizers and a few days off. At that point she came to see me.

In Chinese medicine there is a curious health appraisal known as "empty energy." Using empty energy, people can drive their body to work and worry to the point that only their determination keeps them on their feet. They are all will but with no bodily resources. They drag themselves to work. Shrugging off pain, they stop listening to their bodily feelings. Mrs. Grindhorse bore the symptoms valiantly.

She listened politely to my most persuasive words to rearrange her life and allow her schedule to include daily, systematic rest. I offered her the opportunity to take my classes in stress management. I offered some self-care practices to eliminate pain and balance breathing. But she would have none of it. Her pain belonged to one compartment of her life, her daily obligations to her family and business were something else, far more important than rejuvenation.

How could she even think of taking five minutes out to practice breathing when the business might crumble? To her, rest seemed unethical. She politely refused the offer and breezed through an audit of her behavior and situation, finding nothing in herself that required alteration. She decided to follow the original prescription of drugs and went back to work after a fitful weekend. Three months later she died of heart failure.

Without rest, life's demands become tyrannical.

Without rest, life's demands become tyrannical. Yet busy people put off rest in favor of activity. Some of them view rest as a moral disgrace. They feel guilty if they are not occupying their minds and bodies with busy work. Clever supervisors take advantage of their compulsion, colleagues pay them beautiful compliments for their unrelenting efforts. Some bask in a kind of self-importance and enmeshed identity with their labor. Since their energy is always being exploited, their reserves eventually become depleted. They fail to repay the debt through rest. When their health suffers they become perplexed. Like Charley Brown they ask, "How can this happen when I am so sincere?"

We can appreciate how entrapped they make themselves, but we also need to ask ourselves some serious questions:

- WHAT PREVENTS ME from incorporating restoration as part of my lifestyle?

- DO I GRASP THE IMPORTANCE of rest?

Sometimes, during my work with them, clients let slip some significant statements, that they are sure signs of trouble:

"I feel restless but I can't seem to settle down." Those words are the signal of a life out of control.

"I can't keep up; I must try harder." Hear the compulsion? When I hear that I know the clients' minds impels their bodies beyond capacity. Distress and personal values get mixed together or equated; signals for rest are ignored.

"Who needs rest?" This is usually a signal that the clients put more attention on their ambitions than on their health. They will procrastinate about taking rest since so many other things are more demanding and interesting. "After all," mentioned a friend of mine, "men don't get stressed, they get heart attacks." Their lifestyle sustains a compulsion for stimulation through denial. These people refuse to understand that ambition and health can both be achieved, that the former, in fact, is short-lived without the other.

> "The heart attack did not come out of the blue, as these attacks are supposed to do. The ground was prepared by faulty living and the attack itself was in a way self-induced. This is not mere fancy – it is the result of much reading, inquiry, self-examination and analysis, and careful deduction from known facts.... Stage two on my road back to health was the ability at last to learn to "box clever" – that is, to deal with all stressful conditions, whatever their nature, intelligently and constructively, or else Camille to refuse to have anything to do with them. This implies a degree of mental awareness and self-control which is difficult to cultivate, but which, with perseverance, will always come."[1]
>
> – R. Edwards

Equally subversive are popular "relaxations" undertaken in the spirit of un-stress. Long social hours, an over-filled holiday schedule, entertaining when you need to be alone, weekend partying, can all be draining when you are already tired. The sensual feeling of relaxation, when the energy of wholesome peace and restoration emerges, is simply not possible when a tired body continues to push itself. Learning to say 'no' can be the tonic that heals.

Chronic stress conveys the inadmissible fact that one is using more energy than is being replaced. Obtaining even the best, most nutritious food cannot resolve this predicament; vigorous regular exercise is also not sufficient. There comes an inevitable moment beyond which the body will deteriorate drastically if one does not rest. Even Angels can't help here. Like an alcoholic denying the problem, someone in a recurring state of stress continues to foster self-delusion and the eventual straining of all personal relations.

THE ULTRADIAN RHYTHM

As we have seen in the chapter on breath, the energy flow in our brain and body ordinarily changes every 90 to 120 minutes, correlating with the flow of air through our nostrils. This ultradian cycle is essential to our health. It is nature's reminder to us to take a little rest.

While this healing rhythm is not arbitrary, you can override it.

Many people do – for days, months, even years. The suppression of the ultradian rhythm sets the inexorable conditions for stress-laden illnesses. More dangerously, the neglect of the ultradian rhythm strains one's psychological balance, beckoning belligerence or depression, harassing thoughts of diffidence, and disruptive mood swings. Disregarding the need for rest makes you a loose cannon to yourself and others.

To entertain 15-to-20 minute breaks is not an indulgence but a prime requirement for optimal wellness. Nature provides us with these recurrent, involuntary opportunities to relieve the accumulated stresses in order to enhance our performance of life. Utilizing these periodic rests is like the summer interlude between skiing seasons: one comes back improved from the layoff.

Being active and engrossed in a task eventually comes to a time when the body sends all sorts of signals that a change of pace is eminent. Suddenly, you sense the need for a stretch, or you stare off into space, you get restless, a sigh is felt, attention slightly falters. The crucial moment arrives when you spontaneously notice that your drive is tapering off. At this juncture you have a choice. Either you take a comfort break, allowing the body to rejuvenate itself for renewed performance, or you ignore the signals, driving harder to make up for slipping performance.

The first response acknowledges the natural need for restoration and recharging; the other fosters chronic deterioration in body and mind. The willed efforts to overcome one's natural tiredness or depletion of energy can produce a flush of hormonal hyperactivity that drives one forward with the task at hand. This release of emotional energy can be actually felt and repeatedly aroused in the body. Unfortunately, forced arousal cannot stop the eventual downward spiral in mental performance and emotional composure. A whole gestalt of emotional imbalances will erupt to disfigure the personality and impair judgment. With the latter there is sufficient research to demonstrate that, among other debilitating occurrences over time, the addictive refusal to heed the body's rhythmic call to rest destroys the brain cells of learning and memory.

One's personal ultradian rhythms are not mechanical events showing up at fixed hours. Although the cycle tends to recur approximately every 90–120 minutes, their duration and frequency varies with individuals. The key is to become alert in spotting the biological and mental cues for internal restoration. Acknowledge the periodic comfort response with a brief siesta, a snack, or lie back, fantasize, prolong diaphragmatic breathing and lull yourself into a restorative mood. Figure out your own reconditioning. The cycle's adaptive purpose is to balance your living energy and bring you back to a state of operative wellness for your tasks. Without cooperating with its flexible rhythm there is no chance for maximizing your performance level.

CONSCIOUS REST

Conscious rest enables the body to heal itself. It does for the body what a positive attitude does for the mind. It shifts the direction of your energy from catabolism (expended) to anabolism (renewal). With rest, the body generates energy for conservation, reduces blood pressure and serum cholesterol, and thus promotes recovery. Conscious rest provides wholesome, sensual pleasure and mental satisfaction.

Rest is elusive, however, unless you know how to maximize it. Anyone can sit or lie down for a while and not feel fully restored. The energy of rest is not an illusion nor a waste of time, but neither is it automatically arranged; it requires attention. Conscious rest is an acquired skill.

Your body and brain are a congregation of organic systems in motion. The mind, brain, nervous system and internal organs do not act in mechanical isolation but function organismically. Your autonomic nervous system, endocrine, immune, and neuropeptide systems share a conference call twenty-four hours a day. Whatever seriously affects one, affects all. Body and mind communicate their changing status to each other constantly. Together as conjugate systems they resonate with each other – assuring the maintenance of the ebb and flow of your life energy. The tangible centerpiece of this rhythmic orchestration is breathing. Exhalation and inhalation sustains the orderly flow of energy so that mentally and physically you function from a base of optimum balance.

Stress, coupled with a lack of rest, introduces an interference pattern to the systems. Chronic stress forces strident changes in our emotional and metabolic composure. Intense strain and tiredness reflect a catabolic state in the energy configurations of the mind/body complex. The rhythmic flow of breathing then becomes irregular and consequent aberrations in other systems – muscular tension, irregular heart beat, sweating, nervousness, etc. – produce a feeling of distress. It is this emotional disequilibrium that depletes your energy. If stress is momentary, or the result of healthy exercise, then the systems gradually readjust the metabolic balance. This occurs as long as extreme depletion does not take place. Each of us has a certain tolerance in this regard. Some can put up with more stress interference than others. Your basic outlook on life and its priorities play a crucial role in amplifying or weakening your tolerance.

When interference patterns occur repeatedly, as in emotional swings, or are sustained over long periods of time, such as in brooding and negative thinking, there is a radical change in the relationship among the conjugate systems of the body and mind. Your life energy seems to twist itself out of shape. You feel askew. Non-resonance replaces resonance. The rhythmic entertainment of the systems becomes imbalanced. Illness looms. Along with a host of metabolic dysfunctions burdening your body, many of which may not be evident, (such as high blood pressure, a bleeding ulcer, or a shrinking adrenal gland), the interference pattern signals its degenerative presence by your irregular breath rate. This is the clue to your unstable emotional energy and the reason your customary relaxation remains superficial.

One day a woman came to my office complaining of an inability to relax. Louise said that the feelings of stress were so lodged in her body that she could not remember what it felt like to relax. The word "relax" was an empty abstraction for her. She kept her body in such tension that her entire demeanor was one of aggressive defense toward the world; she felt she had to be on her guard at all times. She experienced life only as the prospect of confrontation. She carried anxiety like a banner. She did not trust drugs and was suspicious of massage.

I told Louise that learning how to relax might compel her to alter some of her attitudes about life. She was willing to give it a try. She laid down as I led her in the practice of progressive relaxation. She was surprised that she liked it, so I sent her home with instructions to perform the exercise once a day, twice if possible.

Louise returned the following week cursing me! On the fifth day of the practice, after about five minutes, she could not feel tension anywhere in her body. The experience of being without her tension terrified her. Although she was in the comfort and safety of her home, she confessed that the more the tension receded the more she felt enormously insecure, fearful, and apprehensive about what dangerous events would happen to her if she continued to relax. She could not allow herself to remain at rest because stresslessness made Louise uncomfortable in dealing with life.

When your anxiety transmits its emotional energy into an irregular breath pattern, your entire person is under siege. Conscious rest in the form of progressive relaxation reverses the depletion of energy, reversing the interference patterns constrained in the muscular tissues. The emergence of uncomfortable feelings and thoughts is not a fault, it is rather the healthy release of stress patterns. When you combine progressive relaxation with diaphragmatic breathing, you induce an energy transition to restoration. Bodily stress wanes as metabolism re-balances. It is this steady recovery of rhythmic balance through attentive breathing that promotes the systemic renewal of energy.

If you can reverse hypertension through systematic breathing, then stress illness can be reversed. Why not allow your body to heal itself? Why set limits to your wellness?

You cannot merely wish for energy; you have to instigate the change to rest and deliberately alter the motion of your energy. Although your nature has innate healing propensities, the habitual condition of degenerate stress may be too advanced for your body to recuperate without deliberate practice.

Unfortunately, for many years physicians have assumed that aging and high blood pressure went hand in hand. They thus declared the aberration of high blood pressure – totally removable – to be normal. While Beta-blocker drugs attempt to mimic the natural control affected by rest, their usefulness is questionable, because they prevent the rested heart rate from growing stronger through exercise.

Diaphragmatic breathing demonstrates its power in affecting

body restoration because it is the optimum norm for homeostatic balance and homeodynamic growth. Progressive relaxation is so powerful because it quickens the mind's communication with the body in order to change those morbid patterns of distress. With the use of these two systematic practices (diaphragmatic breathing and progressive relaxation), older people will find that their natural resistance to tumors and viruses is greatly increased. By bringing posture, breathing and mental attention into alignment, the cycle of energy begins its unimpeded renewal.

Rest is not merely sitting down, playing cards, or watching television. Rest is an art. It must become conscious for its restorative benefits to stabilize. Practice of progressive relaxation and breathing enables the body/mind complex to strengthen its resistance to interference factors. Recuperation is easier, energy reserves are increased, and chronic disease is alleviated. Like all arts, however, rest flourishes from daily, systematic practice.

THE YOGA OF SEEING

Many people have no idea how much the lack of rest affects their eyesight. A well known Wisconsin optometrist, Dr. Ladd Koresch, educates his clients with self-care practices derived from a well-tested, ancient yoga formula in which awareness, breath, and calmness are brought into a unity for better seeing. He has learned from long experiential research how vision reveals the wellness as well as the stresses that one bears. As he educates clients into enhancing the physiological flexibility of their eyes and seeing the actual structures used in the development of visual skills, he encourages them to take an active part in the re-education of their visual skills. With practice, each client gains a perceptive gaze that is free of visual tension. They then see things as they truly are. The clients learn not only to see the surrounding environment but the value and meaning of seeing within.

From our holistic point of view, it should not come as a surprise that our eyes reveal a summary of our general state of health. Most people view their entire body as a collection of separate parts having no essential influence on the well-being of any other part. But when any organ is benefited by rest, exercise, breathing, food, or emotion, the whole share in the benefits.

SLEEP

Sleep is the cure we usually seek when we are tired or exhausted. Sleep assuages physical stress that has accumulated over time. For recovery from severe bouts of chronic stress, sleep is surely the first line of recovery.

We are puzzled, however, when after a night's sleep we wake up tired, sometimes even more tired than when we went to bed. Many of us need drugs to get to sleep at night.[2]

But the inability to fall asleep, fitful sleep, waking up periodically throughout the night, feeling tense in the morning, are not signs that sleep has failed. The lingering tiredness is not coming from sleep but from the body and mind's disposition as we enter the sleep state.

While sleep can bring needful rest to the body, it cannot bring total rest to the mind. When the mind is undergoing disturbance, the quality of sleep is often affected. If you startle yourself out of sleep, it is likely that you carry unresolved tension in the subtle regions of your mind. You then need to examine your lifestyle to illuminate the trouble.

Here is a quick index for identifying embedded stress that affects sleep. An affirmative answer to any of these questions is an indication that stress is chronic.

1. Do I wake up with a start?

2. Do I find it difficult to relax my body?

3. Do I sleep with my mouth open and snore?

4. Do I resist rest even when I do not have to work?

5. Do I find it difficult to be playful with family and friends?

Our wakeful activities use energy – enhancing catabolism – while sleep generates the biological conditions for renewal – anabolism. During sleep, the body repairs itself, allowing for cell division, which normally is diminished during waking hours. Prolonged sleep will help to reestablish energy after trauma. If you have been under a great siege, taking many short naps during the weekend or at the beginning of a vacation is a good idea. Eat lightly and sleep as often as you feel the urge.

PREPARING FOR SLEEP

Although quite natural and apparently automatic, sleep is nevertheless a habit that can be modified. Certain precautions can be taken to assist your body and mind in going to sleep.

1. GO TO BED WITHOUT FOOD.
   Do not eat late at night or just before going to bed. Do not drink cold fluids at night. Ideally, about five hours should pass between your last meal or snack and your sleep. Digestion slows down at night so eating a meal near bedtime puts an extra burden on your internal organs.

2. CALM YOUR EMOTIONS BEFORE YOU SLEEP.
   If you have recently been involved in either an emotionally enthralling or particularly negative experience, wait awhile until your feelings to calm before trying to sleep. Otherwise you may spend hours repeating the episode.

3. DISTRACT YOUR MIND.
   If you find yourself reliving events of the past or pondering the future over and over, then it might be better to distract your mind by getting up and reading for awhile. Don't, however, choose a book so intriguing that it captures your attention and keeps you awake!

4. HAVE A BRIEF DIALOGUE WITH YOUR MIND.
   Tell your mind that while the items it brings up are important, you will attend to them tomorrow. Respond that it should allow your body to slumber so that you can be refreshed and ready to consider those very items the next day.

5. BREATHE AWAY MENTAL CONGESTION WITH DIAPHRAGMATIC BREATHING.

PRACTICE SESSION

Get to Sleep

Here is a secret method for getting to sleep:

- LIE DOWN on your back with your arms extended along your sides but slightly away from your body.

- CLOSE YOUR EYES and mouth.

- NOW ASK YOUR BODY to be still.

- BEGIN TO EXHALE more deeply with some attention and let your inhalation take place without forcing it.

- YOUR ABDOMINAL AREA will flatten or move downwards as you exhale, and rise upwards as you inhale.

- YOUR BREATHING should be gentle and without strain.

- ALLOW YOUR BREATHING to become smooth and quiet, without jerks in the flow of breath.

- ALLOW THIS EXHALATION/INHALATION to occur for 8 breaths.

- ON YOUR NEXT EXHALATION feel as though your exhalation is slowly moving from the crown of your head downwards through your body and out your toes.

- YOUR INHALATION moves slowly from your toes upwards through your body and out the crown.

- DO THIS MOTION of breathing gently, allowing the mind to move along with the direction of the breath.

- DO THIS TEN TIMES and then roll over unto your left side.

- BREATHE 15 TIMES on your left side.

- ROLL OVER GENTLY to your right side.

- BREATHE 30 TIMES on your right side.

- SWEET DREAMS!

NOTE: This exercise is available on cassette tape; see order page.

Solitude:
Discover the World Within

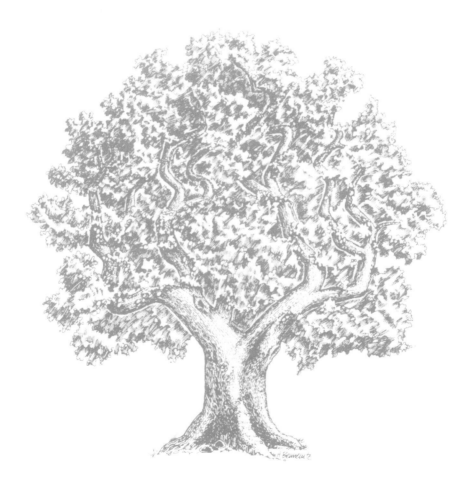

HUMAN BEINGS have a need to share energy in some way with one another. For this reason we form clubs, teams, committees, institutes. Community is one of the most important features of life. Whether it is a vibrant family or a dynamic company, positive collective effort is always required to sustain the group. This measure of the collective effort directly bears upon the personal mastery of each individual. While communities need one another to act for a common purpose, it is equally important to acknowledge the source of each individual's personal power. The empowering root of personal mastery is solitude.

ONLY THE SILENT SEE

Solitude is a part of life that is often neglected and consequently goes unappreciated. We have a profound need to be alone just as we have a need for community. The art of solitude has a long history of practitioners who were, through their art, able to gain a healthier perspective on life. Until the joys of being alone with oneself are experienced, however, it is difficult to imagine how wonderful solitude can be.

For many of us, devising time to be alone takes a great deal of cleverness. With a demanding career, family claims and an active social life, arranging for solitude takes Machiavellian inspiration. Yet there should be moments where the cares and duties of the world are put aside, where one can enter a space in which no one else trespasses, where one can be alone, but not lonely.

To speak of solitude in this way is reminiscent of monasteries and convents. There the quiet environment provides a background for introspective practices requiring solitude, and so it is enforced. But with planning and a little luck solitude can be practiced anywhere. It is more in the mind than in the environment, although a quiet atmosphere is certainly conducive to exploration of the inner world.

Solitude is the most intense opportunity for pursuing the meaning of self. Even those specific relationships with others that we experience as unique and irreplaceable, that give our life its social significance, cannot provide us with the self-discovery and replenishing knowledge that the intimacy of solitude does. It gives us a sense of being whole.

Andre Malraux wrote of the painter Goya, "To allow his genius to become apparent to himself it was necessary that he should dare to give up aiming to please."[1] So much of our life is governed by reactions to others; we judge ourselves by how others judge us. In the privacy of solitude, however, we can gain the uninfluenced knowledge of ourselves that is true and necessary. In solitude, we are on our own. No pressure. Nobody watching.

One of the main reasons we neglect solitude is because we resist intimacy with ourselves. Sometimes we pretend that solitude is boring, but actually we find being alone uncomfortable. Our minds taunt us when we are alone, away from our ordinary occupations and distractions. We are too easily reminded of what we do not like about ourselves. Why should we bother to increase that pain? Our environment provides sufficient criticism without rehearsing it again in solitude. Perhaps.

THE GAZE THAT RENEWS

A nurse worked in the terminal ward of a London hospital, constantly dealing with physical and emotional forms of disintegration and death. Although she had been working in that busy ward for several years, there was a sensitive calmness about her that stirred my curiosity. On one visit, I asked how she coped daily with a environment where fear, anger, despair, and death prevailed. Her answer was curious. Not too many years ago, she purchased a small cottage in one of those picturesque English country villages where even time forgets its mission. Most weekends would find her there, sitting in the garden, facing the westerly landscape, surrounded by her sunlit companions – the abundant flowers, trees, shrubs – and listening to the sounds from the surrounding forest. In the quiet enchantment of those hours, she gazed upon the living forces of nature. Within the solitude of her retreat, she contemplated beauty: she experienced the vision that renews.

Contemplation nourishes the energy of the human spirit by putting it back into touch with the primal truths of life. Most of life is monopolized by domestic and commercial enterprises. They pay the bills, keep the house tidy, and secure our place in society. But our spirit longs for more than duty, more than paying the mortgage.

Nature is in our blood and we need to respond to her summons. Pack a lunch and spend a day in the country or by the seashore. Wandering aimlessly over the terrain, letting your senses alight upon natural surroundings that are not routine, produces a restoration that is impossible to duplicate any other way.

If the sea or the woods are too far away, find a special time and place that brings you back home alone with yourself, an oasis of solitude where you can incidentally relieve your accumulated stresses. Listening to your favorite music, enjoying a hobby, exploring a new neighborhood, composing poetry, strolling alone through the cool night air under the stars – these are the contemplative moments that stir and heal, that revive your lagging energy, that show you that life offers more than your worries.

In 1983 the Nobel prize was awarded to eighty-one-year-old Barbara McClintock for her discoveries in gene research. Much of her work was done on the corn plant. Her intimate knowledge of the plants came from going into the fields and being with the corn. Through her contemplation she developed a "feeling" for the organism. The special time of gazing upon the living organisms enriched her understanding: "I don't feel I really know the story if I don't watch the plant all the way along … hear what the material has to say to me, let it come to me.... I have learned so much about the corn plant that when I see things, I can interpret them right away."[2]

This contemplative feeling enabled Barbara to penetrate many of the secrets of genes unsuspected in scientific circles. Her biographer says: "So adept did she become at recognizing the outward signs of those structural alterations in chromosomal composition that she could simply look at the plants themselves and know what the microscopic inspection of the cells' nuclei would later reveal."[3] Her hours of contemplation eventually evoked a process of creative insight that rational analysis later confirmed through lengthy laboratory procedures. "When you suddenly see the problem, then something happens and you have the answer – before you are able to put it into words. It is all done subconsciously. This has happened too many times to me, and I know when to take it seriously."[4]

Even as an undergraduate student, it was evident that McClintock had a capacity for total absorption in her subject and an ability to become one with the object of her contemplation. She often said she would like to forget her body and just be with the reality at hand. During one geology examination, her absorption in the subject was the cause of embarrassment. McClintock states that she loved the subject so much that there was nothing that could be asked in the exam that she did not know already. Her delight in writing out and finishing the exam came to an abrupt stop at the end of the page: she could not remember her name! She anguished for minutes until finally she remembered it.

McClintock possessed a reverence for the mysterious intricacies of nature as well as the awesome power of the mind. Later in life she became interested in Eastern methods of learning, impressed by the Himalayan yogis' ability to regulate body temperature. She asserts, "We are scientists, and yet we know basically nothing about controlling our body temperature. The Tibetans learn to live with nothing but a tiny cotton jacket. They're out there in cold winters and hot summers, and when they have been through the learning process, they have to take certain tests. One of the tests is to take a wet blanket, put it over them, and dry that blanket in the coldest weather. And they dry it."[5]

Barbara McClintock herself is an endangered species, a rare genre of scientist who insists that conventional science is in default unless it includes the act of contemplation in its methodology. If scientists want to really read the text of nature, then they must "take the time and look." They must enter solitude.

The artificial constraints of schedule, overwork, and allegiance to "busy-ness" entwine your soul fiercely. They keep you from realizing your life force and tapping its energy. How can you get back in touch with your own vital force?

In ancient Greece, the theater was used as therapy to confront the problems of spirit and become healed. You can enter solitude as the Greeks entered the theater.

Like so many others, you have become wearied by the stresses of living. Your hidden burden of stale joys and regret is not unlike that of others who are joining you as tired members of society. You enter the theater like enrolling for a retreat. You are escorted to sit and watch. Upon the stage a drama begins and engages your questioning self. You wonder whether you made the right choice in coming. What does it matter? Nothing works anymore.

Accompanied by your cynical doubts, you listen and watch, resisting, yet drawn into the action. Is it possible that the woeful tale echoes your own plight? How curious. Your wandering attention lessens. Interest heightens. You think it impossible, but the players become a projection of your struggles. You are engaged, challenged to cast your lot with them. The emotional polarities of the scenes acknowledge your own conflicting reactions to life's unfair predicaments. "Listen," they seem to say, "life is like this for everyone."

Feeling for the characters, you reflect their consternation in yourself. Seething with empathy, you weep and laugh at their recognizable foibles, and suffer their struggling lives through your own mind and heart, until finally the story resolves itself not only upon the theater floor but, incredibly, upon the stage of your soul.

What appears a theater becomes a temple of revelation. You endure a catharsis. Purified from the gnarled energy of ingrown resentment and melancholy, you awake to the truthful passions of life's story. Your familiar, tormenting emotions are burst wide open from their insufferable boundaries of anxiety and diffidence that had fatigued you for years. The past is past. Shorn of self-incrimination and old pity, your freed spirit revives its self-awareness once more with the assuring strength of being alive with promise. Healing moves swiftly throughout your wrinkled body and now enlarged mind. Hope tremors your thoughts. A fresh vision of life's worth resumes its course. Torn order is mended. There is beauty upon the earth. You feel astonished. More centered, a little wiser than when you came in, you exit into the world. *Contemplation made you whole again.*[6]

Unless your daily life occasionally astounds you into a more profound context than the entropy of culture gossip, the human spirit will smother. The passing truths of our work-a-day world give us some reflection, but they are utterly insufficient to nourish our higher dreams. If all your spirit imbues is Muzak, U.S.A. *Today*, internet surfing, and sit-coms, it suffers anemia. Occasionally we need those experiences that take us beyond the obvious, beyond the most common denominator, beyond the immediate schedules of our private and political lives.

According to Plato's reflections, each of us summarizes the universe in all its order and chaos. In our personal odyssey through life, we uniquely replay the grand themes of creation and history, growth and dissolution. But like a phoenix, our spirit is meant to shed its illusions, to rise again and again from the ashes of our evolving drama in order to come closer to the imperishable center of our being. We are, after all, spiritual beings moving through time and space, testing life, undergoing human experiences to resolve our quest for the Tree of Life.

THE THERAPY OF SUFFERING

There are certain intimate moments we should savor before coming to the end of life. When the conditions are right, we will have epiphanies that help us rediscover the light and strength sorely missing in our daily lives. We cannot grab or hoard those experiences; we can only enjoy them and then draw upon their power for our journey.

We see in silence.

We see in silence. Without the encounter of profound truth, there is no experience of beauty; without the sheen of beauty there is no contemplation; without contemplation we wander lost in an oppressive, meaningless world, feeling only its unpredictable chaos. This is why it is so important to attempt the right setting, to assume the right frame of mind. Hence the awesome role of suffering.

We all understandably shun discomfort. Suffering, however, forces its own healthy dialectics; it arouses self-questioning. Why me? Why so often? What did I do to deserve this? Reassessing ourselves, we confront the truth and its painful consequences: If I do not clear up my act, I am doomed to repeat it. Yet repeat it we do; we postpone reality again and again.

Finally, one weary day, the soul balks; it is tired of getting what is has always gotten: lopsided truths with short careers. Enough is enough. The time is ripe. Whether you suspect it or not, you are dangerously near an astonishing event: the breaking of spells. Society has cast its own allurements of thin beauty upon you; you yourself have made other mirages by clinging to narrow ideas, shredding your emotions over the past, inviting a host of doubts and recriminations, refusing to reorder your life. Now you taste the desolation. The moment has come for you. Your spirit shrieks out, tired of merely scraping through life. Like the Eskimo in the wilderness, you lament:

> But where did my soul go?
> Come home, come home.

You finally recognize that you feel powerless amidst temporary schemes because you neglected richer truths. Yet for all your neglect of her bounty, life is not spiteful. In this awesome condition you are ready to enter the mindset where a great gift is possible. Life awaits your failure so that she can grant you her boon – calling you to exceed your withered dreams. Follow your lament unto a new landscape where the tree of life grows. There you will learn to drop your comforting self-pity. Your wounds hurt, but they have brought your heart into a silence where a new, corrective vision stirs into focus. Without the almost unbearable pain, you would not have stretched your spirit to enter this new covenant with life. There, among its many disclosures, life shows you through the quiet act of contemplation how to heal and reorder your entire life force. What regulated breathing does for your bodily systems, so gazing upon the radiance of life does for your spirit. Contemplation is the healing gift that enlivens.

INNER JOURNEY TO WHOLENESS

Meditation is another art that revives and expands life. It may be described as a quieting of the mind and body so that conscious tranquillity and rational clarity may emerge. Whereas the gaze of contemplation is outward bound, resting upon the beauty and power of the manifested universe, the gaze of meditation is inward, dwelling upon the silent, enriching galaxies of the spirit.

In meditation's moments of quiet renewal, you also step aside from the busy routine of schedules, paying bills, phone calls. You are reclusive for a while; you retire from the structures of time. For this reason, meditation is sometimes thought of as an escape from life to enter the timeless place where renewal takes place. Meditation can be abused as a form of escape, but its true nature is vastly superior to escape.

Often the words 'contemplation' and 'meditation' are cast incorrectly. They have become associated with a definite religious pattern of living. In themselves, however, neither one is a religious practice. While sometimes connected to prayer, contemplation and meditation are more akin to personal hygiene – wholly natural ways to touch your life force at a deeper awareness than the ever-changing surfaces that compel your daily occupation.

Meditation is a direct solitary journey into your life energy. No companions are allowed. The senses systemically stilled, you enter, quietly through the portals of your busy mind into its underlying hidden consciousness, there to dwell upon the life force alone. You embark without aggression, without the compensation of thoughts because the deeper domains of life will not be intimidated by coercion or competition. You cannot bully your spirit to comply with your mission. You sit, as the medieval text of the *Cloud of Unknowing* relates[7] with a "naked intent," seeking within the wellsprings of life. All your beliefs are left behind. Meditation feels its way by inner awareness to the vast silent domain of your unblemished spirit. In that homeland of incredible power and beauty, all loneliness vanishes.

For a long while meditation proceeds more at the biological level, inducing relaxation and reducing stress. These are tremendous boons that need to be acquired before one advances further. The subtle powers of the mind opens its immortal treasures only when mind and body have achieved a certain integration through dynamic rest. Once relaxation spreads throughout your person, then your mind can release its concern for the body and its memories and proceed on its way.

If you were to use meditation only in terms of a basic hygiene, you could practice it for ten to fifteen minutes on a daily basis. This practice alone would have the healthful effects of enabling you to cope more easily with the customary stress encountered in your daily occupations. But meditation beckons you to much more; it can introduce you to yourself.

MEDITATION MENTOR

The rudiments of meditation can be learned in a short time. From then on, the development of the skill is a matter of subtle persistence. In meditation, however, as in life, a mentor is a great help. For those who sincerely desire to pursue the depths of meditation, a skilled mentor is indispensable. Your mentor or tutor should have a great deal of experience with life, a lifestyle consistent with meditation, and many years' experience in practicing the art.

In meditation, you will meet mind adventures, not all of which are simple to successfully navigate. Has your teacher prepared you for them? From the fertile regions of your consciousness come both adversaries and allies to test your endeavor. Your progress eventually summons the demons of fantasy from your chamber of memories. You have to slay the dragons of distraction, boredom, suppressed emotions, unrealized desires, not because they are obnoxious, but to prove to yourself that their energy patterns are less then you deserve. You are meant for more than the sensory and intellectual properties of this planet. If you build your endurance of spirit through meditation you eventually rediscover your forgotten inheritance: you are a citizen of the entire universe laying claim to your homeland.

Sometimes meditators get caught when intuition opens and psychic phenomena occurs. These are natural products of interior work. While no power of the mind should be left unintegrated, no idea is so precious and profitable that it can define who you are. The power of meditation lies in gradually releasing the subtle hold that the contents of your mind and heart have over you. You do not banish them so much as recast their importance. With your identity in healthy perspective, you can direct your life force to greater unfoldment. You step into a landscape called freedom. The mentor then assists you in keeping poised in the expanding context of your adventure.

Meditation sets the scene for an inner healthy transformation of the complexities of your personal consciousness. Over time, a creative reorganization of your inner, experiential life leads to more positive, responsible behavior. A Roshi whom I knew once remarked that after reaching his enlightenment, he still went to the bathroom, but now measured the toilet paper. His awareness was such that he was now always in alignment with life. Meditation inspires your conduct: the expression of energy without becomes consistent with the energy within. You are less willing to be deceived by careless motives. When you are in touch with yourself, reality has a clearer ring to it. With purer eyes, the dissembling of others is easily seen: there you were but a short time ago. Through these awakening episodes, you recognize stages of ripening in yourself.

In the dark solitude of meditation, your eyes are opening, perhaps for the first time, to the amazing discrepancies in the world at large – personal, social, political. These revelations can be traumatic. Again, the mentor aids in clarification: it is not a perfect, but a perfectible world. Slowly, organically, your spirit acquires the endurance it needs for the tasks of life ahead.

You say your goal is nothing less than the secrets of the universe? Meditation acquires the skills of the spirit for that long journey. When you gather your mind and heart in the cloak of silence, you awaken the invincible force that conquers all inner obstacles, all the stumbling blocks that your history has bequeathed to you. Your future yields only to the power of silence. Let it become an effortless witnessing.

MEDITATION AND THE BODY

Meditation has a profound influence on your personality. The slow, subtle breathing, the resting posture, the focused attention, gradually releases the stress-bound energy of your memory patterns, enabling you to balance your attitude. With these patterns in harmony, a new feeling of peaceful centering occurs. During meditation practice, the energy resonance of mind and body waxes and wanes heading into the theta range of brain activity. A poised awareness emerges, which approximates the "normal" setting for humans.[8] For as a silent witness, you discover that your mind can remain unchangeable amidst its fluctuations of thought, image, and feeling. You can easily feel the difference before and after your practice.

For the past forty years, meditation has been repeatedly researched for its clinical and therapeutic benefits. It has been implicated in reducing a range of stress-related dysfunctions from headaches and hypertension to diabetes and cancer. Some researchers consider meditation the most positive antidote for preventing and alleviating prolonged stress responses.

Our most pernicious stresses lie hidden within us. We bury them in our memories, but, regretfully, they are not deceased; they merely act outside normal rational awareness. Like important but unfinished business, the incidence of dysfunctional behavioral patterns and rational suppression accumulates in our bodies. Their pangs of distress are tolerated, anesthetized, or marginalized by the pressure of our immediate goals. In our everyday, rational awareness, we can disassociate from these uncomfortable patterns by retiring them into the store house of our memories. Unfortunately they do not remain inactive in storage. On the contrary, their invisible but dynamic presence colors our everyday thinking, is felt in the occasional acute crisis, or in the general rundown feeling associated with entropy and old age. In any case, their warnings for the future are often ignored.

Emotional stress accumulates in one's memory without showing up in an obvious, forthright manner, like a decent headache, for example. You know when someone bumps you because you feel the pressure. The culprit of stress is not always that obvious. The memory of stress experiences lurk in you, but not merely as idea. Even when there is no constant dramatic crisis, the stress-bound memory patterns constrain your life force. Like hypertension, which can be habitually present in the body but unfelt in the mind, these unconscious patterns have a noxious effect on your metabolism as well as your outlook.

Stress-bound patterns build up from your unresolved lifestyle episodes and work habits. The original stressful experience you struggled through is not a mental abstraction but an occurrence that was felt in your body. There is a visceral and emotional association with the mental scene. You – mind and body, thought and cell – undergo the charged experience. Like other memories, this stored energy of the event is retained, encoded as a cellular memory.

Thus your memories indicate not just an eventful idea undergone in the past, but encapsulated information-as-energy, making the unresolved past a living force in the present. On this basis the roots of chronic stress stay hidden as confined memories that subliminally impede your well-being. There are many bodily ailments connected with these embedded cellular memories that do not signal severe distress for months, even years, and yet daily take their corrosive toll. Ulcers, arthritis, tremors, cataracts, surfacing bouts of uncontrolled negative thinking, a general anxiety about the future, unpaid vendettas, a simmering hostility towards certain people – all held in check, of course, but active nevertheless – are just some of the constraining information patterns that nest in your person. These unattended negative memories are entropic stress patterns that ill-shape the dynamics of human living.

FORMS OF MEDITATION

There are many forms of meditation; some are associated with particular cultures and others have religious overtones.[9] Meditation in itself, however, is a dynamic of human nature and can be understood and practiced purely as a way of becoming still so that body, mind, and spirit renew themselves in an exalted way.

When your mind is agitated, it is impossible for you to feel relaxed. Your body always mirrors your thoughts. Likewise, when your mind is calmly directed toward your goals, your body tends to be equally supportive. Hence the importance of a practice that aligns your entire person.

Meditation attempts to improve this integration by expanding your self-awareness. By calmly paying attention to your stream of thoughts, images and feelings, without getting either upset by them nor actively curious about their presence, you begin to gain a wider perspective toward the colorful contents of your mind. The stream of contents entertains as well as bores. In meditation, you learn how not to be compelled by the mind's configuring energy. Thus, in reaching the balanced state of energy between mind and body, you strengthen your body's efforts to heal itself from its imbalances.

Worry and anxiety are very similar to meditation, except that they are its obverse. Worry constricts, hurts, and depletes energy; meditation expands, heals, stimulates the life force. Worry drains your attention and thus prevents you from using other avenues of response to the problem. You become so engrossed with your anxiety that you are unable to see the possibilities for resolving the predicament even when they are obvious. Worry and meditation both are one-pointed concentration; the former contracts the person while the latter expands the awareness of life.

The internal chatter of the mind tends to be wayward, exploiting your energy in random bursts. Anxiety keeps you vulnerable to incidentals: it follows the opinions and whims from the external world. Your attention jumps from one thought to another, from considering this to considering that, arousing unregulated emotion with each jump. These distractions interfere with your concentration. You feel frustrated by the interruptions and later brood about them endlessly. Anxiety wearies the nervous system; its incessant arousal wears down the body and fixates attention. Worry yields a negative trance that lowers vitality.

Meditation, on the contrary, stimulates the parasympathetic nervous system and inhibits the hyper-arousal of the worry response. The inevitable stillness is not lethargy, but renewal. Meditation is, by far, the most powerful self-care resource you possess. Through the resource of meditation, you can:

- PUT LIFE'S EPISODES into a balanced context,

- GAIN MASTERY over your attention,

- OPEN THE DOOR to intuitive awareness.

Your self-understanding widens from the trees to the forest. Instead of getting emotionally transfixed by your problems, meditation calms your energy, enabling your mind to view problems in a broader context, and then see their solution.

In meditation, you learn to pay attention by an easy, direct, steady gaze. Rhythmic breathing and gentle focusing coordinate, allowing the mind to dissociate from its agitating thought patterns. Mental and emotional restoration stirs. It takes awhile before the mind accustoms itself to being in solitude, but once it does, it will savor it. It is like realizing a treasure of calm energy that you did not know existed.

Patience is needed for meditation. The mind likes to skip around on various thoughts and images. To help in the beginning, the meditator focuses attention upon a designated object. This object is not arbitrarily chosen. It can be the act of breathing itself, a special sound, or a certain figure. Actually, your calm, breathing rhythm aids enormously in settling your mind's attention. The objective here is not to restrict thinking but to direct the mind's energy in a single gaze. As time goes on, the thoughts and images that emerge will have less and less power to distract you from your inward journey.

As you gain ascendancy over your concentrated inward gaze, the calming of your nervous system and the growing stillness of your mind become more pronounced, allowing the subtle, healing benefits of meditation to unfold.

Among the many physiological benefits recorded in meditational research are:

- A 50 PERCENT OR MORE DECREASE IN RESPIRATORY RATE.
  In meditation, body metabolism slows down even more than when in sleep. Consequently, the internal systems of the body derive profound rest and the metabolism regenerates itself, forestalling the aging processes.

- IMPROVED DILATION OF PERIPHERAL BLOOD VESSELS.
  This change in blood vessel dilation indicates muscular relaxation. Illness, such as migraine headaches and Raynaud's disease can thus be reversed.[10]

- CONTROL OVER EMOTIONAL AROUSAL IS IMPROVED.
  Repeated practice of meditation produces a qualitative improvement in alertness to personal environment. This growth in awareness enables one to remain less disturbed, even relaxed, in the presence of inhibiting stress activity. As a result of inducing a more relaxed internal state, including a reduced heart rate, metabolic stability is fos-

tered. Even amidst acute disturbances, the accumulated effects of daily meditation promote easier recovery, which is normally difficult for those with chronic anxiety.

People can become so disrupted by stress responses over the years that the mind-body complex finds it virtually impossible to rebound into relaxation. Meditation offers a resource for retraining individual responses toward a sense of balanced living. As you progress in the art, you become more alert and responsible without being tense. Your normal awareness of yourself – your feelings and thoughts about relationships, your employment, state of health, relationships, etc. – undergoes a change. Your personal investment of time and energy in these areas becomes much more obvious to you. Concentration improves. The overall sense of what you are doing with your life becomes more apparent. You are more able to make positive goals and match your actions to those goals. You become able to make decisions about what and who are important in your life. Before, in the pursuit of your goals, you would ignore or override the stress signals that crept up as you were completing your tasks. You would squander time. Now you detect tension at its beginning stages. This increased awareness leads to the courage to make appropriate necessary changes that will make your life more fulfilling.

In a world of high tech attractions and so many drugs, it seems strange to propose that the process of stilling the body and mind through contemplation and meditation promotes such profound renewal. But we cannot truly know reality and gain our own power over our mind-body health unless we practice the art of solitude.

PRACTICE SESSION

When we want to learn something new about our work we give it our full attention. The same is true when we want to learn about ourselves. The attention of our senses is imperative, because that is the chief way we bring our environment inside. Let's try an experiment.

Experiment I: Expanding Sense Awareness

🍂 CHOOSE A SPOT in the woods and sit there for a half hour. Patiently follow these sequences to expand your senses, and keep your attention fully alert to the specific sense. If your mind drifts off, gently bring it back to that sense.

🍂 FIRST, CLOSE YOUR EYES, calm your breath, and just listen to the environment. Listen with the idea that you are extending your hearing: in front, at your sides, behind, above, below. Be receptive to all sounds; hear the sounds close to you and the sounds far away. Listen for five minutes.

🍂 WITHOUT OPENING YOUR EYES, pay attention to your sense of smell. Extend your awareness to all the scents in your environment for five minutes.

🍂 CONTINUE YOUR ATTENTION but shift it to your tongue for discerning various tastes that linger there. Open you mouth slightly and note the tastes that are carried on the air.

🍂 NOW OPEN YOUR EYES and for five minutes look around in all directions, carefully, slowly, absorbing the environment both near and far through your eyes.

🍂 NEXT, FOR FIVE MINUTES feel the atmosphere with the kinesthetic sense of your skin. Note the temperature, the touch of the wind, pressure under your legs and feet, the touch of an insect, the weight of the humidity. Remain sitting peacefully while you feel your environment.

🍂 FINALLY BECOME AWARE of your total environment with all your senses at once. Sit for five minutes listening, smelling, tasting, seeing, and feeling.

🍂 HOW DO YOU FEEL about yourself now? About nature? Any new insights?

Experiment II: Inner Renewal of Meditation

- CHOOSE A TIME when you can have ten to twenty minutes of uninterrupted quiet. A good time might be very early in the morning or late at night. Turn off your phone, close your door, and ask that you not be disturbed.

- LIE DOWN or sit in a comfortable chair so that your head, neck and trunk can be upright without being rigid. Place your hands on your thighs if you are sitting, or turn them palms up if you are lying down.

- CLOSE YOUR EYES and mouth.

- DO ONE SERIES of alternate nostril breathing as found in Chapter 3: Breath. Keep your attention on the exchange of inhalation and exhalation as it enters each nostril.

- NOW CONCENTRATE on the practice of diaphragmatic breathing for a few breaths.

- NEXT, PERFORM THE PRACTICE of progressive relaxation, as described in Chapter 2: Attitude. Proceed slowly and carefully, including all the major areas of the body.

- EXHALE AND INHALE from the crown of your head to your toes and back again for five breaths. Each breath should be slow, deliberate, careful, restful. Take your time.

- NOW BEGIN TO SHORTEN the flow of your breath by exhaling from the crown of your head to your ankles.

    Inhale and exhale from the crown to your knees.

    Inhale and exhale from your crown to the base of your spine.

    Inhale and exhale from the crown to your bladder.

    Inhale and exhale from the crown to your solar plexus.

    Inhale and exhale from the crown to the center of your chest.

    Inhale and exhale from the crown to your throat pit.

Inhale and exhale from the crown to the small junction between your nostrils where you can feel the cool air coming into your nostrils and the warm air going out.

- AFTER A FEW MINUTES allow your attention to rise to the space between your eyebrows. Rest your attention there and allow your breathing to continue smoothly and continuously. Gradually it will slow down and become very calm.

- WHATEVER THOUGHTS, images, or feelings come before your memory, simply observe them without becoming committed to them.

- IF YOU GET DISTRACTED by the thoughts, just return your attention to your breathing. Let your breathing become the object of your attention.

- STAY HERE and enjoy the silence.

- WHEN YOU WOULD LIKE to end the practice, expand your breath throughout your body, gently move your fingers and toes, remember where you are sitting or lying, open your eyes, and rise slowly and gently.

    NOTE: This meditational practice is available on cassette tape in *Wellness Tree Tapes*; see order page.

PART 3

THE TRUNK
OF POSSIBILITIES

CHAPTER 8

Choosing Life

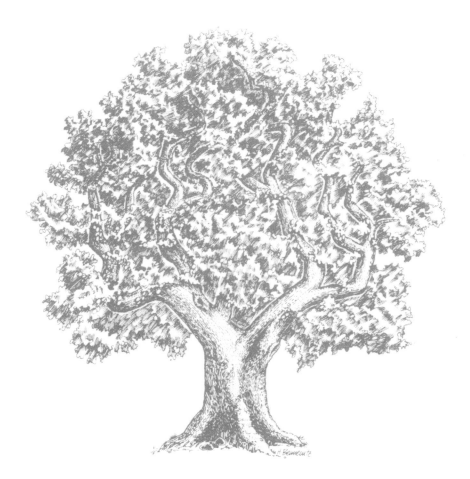

Many years ago a new village was deeded a large grove of fruit trees. At first the village inhabitants walked and played in the grove, celebrating the seasons under its leafy branches. They enjoyed and admired the forest, and took good care of the trees, but they never touched its magnificent fruit.

As the town folk became older and less energetic, raking and pruning the grove proved too much work for them. So they erected a high fence around the trees and put up a shiny new sign on it: "Forbidden to enter." Now they would not have to clear the area for walking or picnicking. They could admire the beauty of the trees from afar.

Totally unknown to the aging village people was the power of the fruit on the trees. It contained all the energy that they needed to restore their vitality and extend their lives. Now, alas, the trees with the gift of life were off-limits.

It was not long before the village completely forgot about the fruit grove, and its celebrations faded from memory. In the last news from that place, it was suggested that the old clump of trees might make saleable lumber.

We are like those village people. We get so caught up with our private aspirations and public obligations that we forget our continual dependence on the energy of life. We occupy our minds with tasks requiring energy, but seldom pause to consider what it actually is that keeps us alive. In our rush to succeed in one area of life, we become careless about renewing our energy for the others. We eat poorly and on the run; we subject our bodies to a great deal of strain with insufficient rest; we allow brooding thoughts to weaken our metabolism, agitate emotions, and dilute sleep. Instead of mastering life for greater enjoyment, we grope with life's challenges and find our lives discordant.

Life's vast energy for strength, intelligence, peace and joy is always there. Yet as long as we take the life force for granted, we use only a small portion of it. Whether you are ill or well, whether you want more or less, your attitude toward life's force is crucial for accessing its energy. The resource for either option is the same: the vitality of the mind.

Along with concepts and ideas that we form about ourselves, we have another faculty that plays an essential role in association with our thoughts and emotions. That is the power of imagination. Since the energy of imagination interfaces with the mind and body, we can generate images that both symbolize and modify the way we feel and think. Tinkering with imagery can aid us in revealing aspects of ourselves that may escape mere conceptualization.

Who would suppose that a concentrated, positive intent, imaginatively conceived and accompanied by a cheerful enthusiasm, could drastically alter the immunological factors composing the blood? Well, it has already been proven.

Within a laboratory setting, Norman Cousins of UCLA's School of Medicine pondered the unusual idea of a joint United States and Russian foreign policy. He thought about all the world's benefits if such a mutually designed, rational, humanitarian program were implemented. While he thought this positive thought, he felt the mounting flush of euphoria that the scenario provoked in his body. After five minutes of this concentration, his blood showed an increase of fifty-three per cent in the number of cells in his immune system. In fact, the antibody-coated T-cells showed a two hundred per cent increase.[1] Who knows what he could have generated in his immune system if he had imagined a settlement of the Middle East crisis!

In the midst of other scientific experiments at the Menninger Foundation, Swami Rama of the Himalayas, a visiting consultant, spontaneously produced two cysts on his body, one on each forearm. A biopsy was immediately performed on each. The report on the tissues confirmed his prediction: on one forearm the cyst was benign, on the other, cancerous. After the biopsies, the consultant immediately dissolved the two growths, leaving smooth skin.[2]

Numerous such reports, clinical as well as anecdotal, are available for those who need corroborative evidence that mind and matter are such close companions that they can hardly refuse one another any request.

HOW MUCH LIFE DO YOU WANT?

What request do you have for your own mind-body? The majority of us would like better health and more energy. Everyone talks about feeling better, but for many of us talk is about as far as it goes. Some of us easily gloss over our well being until a crisis strikes; then suddenly the recovery of vitality is a most stern affair. Once we are well again, our concern for life's energy recedes farther and farther from daily patterns into forgetfulness – until another crisis arrives. Unless a catastrophe scares us, we do not pay much attention to how we are utilizing the energy of our bodies and minds.

At this moment you are obviously alive, but consider these questions carefully:

- Do you want to feel more alive?

- Do you want to enrich yourself with more of life's energy?

- Do you know how to call upon unlimited energy resources for renewal?

- Would you like to be less susceptible to tiredness, chronic stress, and illness?

- Do you want to exert more bodily vigor and be less tired while you work?

- What would having more vitality mean for you?

By more vitality I do not mean the feeling you have after taking aspirin to relieve a headache or the feeling you get after a much-needed massage. These feelings are relief. I am also not referring to the result of building a girth of muscles, or losing those extra twenty pounds you carry around. What I do mean is having natural energy resources available whenever you want them. Would you say such resources were priceless? Undoubtedly. But there is a catch. To claim your energy you have to ask for it!

In my pursuit of optimal wellness, I observed four things about human beings that surprised and saddened me. After many years of observing and talking with people in Europe, the British Isles, the Middle East, India, Japan, and the United States, I reluctantly admit:

🖋 MOST PEOPLE CHOOSE FOR THEMSELVES A CONDITION OF LIFE THAT IS LESS THAN WELL.

People are not particularly aware of this choice. They are ordinary citizens or professional leaders, poor or wealthy, educated or not. They have their good days and their bad ones and they accept their ups and downs as the normal routine of life. They complain little because their colds, flu, aches, and pains come and go with only an occasional serious disorder. They think robust wellness might be for Olympic athletes; they do not think it can ever be for them.

🖋 MOST PEOPLE EXPECT MORE AND MORE ILLNESS IN THEIR FUTURE.

They assume that as they get older and slow down, their wellness will decline and they will get worse. That's what happened to their parents, so it will happen to them. They think it's the acceptable way to age. They accept the inevitable; in fact they expect it and plan for it.

🖋 MOST PEOPLE DO NOT THINK THEY CAN GET WELL WITHOUT DRUGS OR SURGERY.

When these people were shown how to upgrade their vitality without depending upon any external medication, their smiling disbelief showed that they regarded the evidence to be far-fetched. They politely informed me that since none of their friends could upgrade their health, how could they? Their reasons for avoiding the possibility of such a change were breathtaking.

🖋 THOSE WHO ACCEPTED THE IDEA OF OPTIMUM WELLNESS SOON DISCOVERED THAT THEY COULD DO WHAT ONCE BELONGED TO YOUTH ALONE.

When some of the people decided to try self-care and persisted in self-care practices, they found they could reverse tired feelings, eliminate chronic illness, and create new possibilities with their energy resources.

If you are less well than you want to be, if you feel up one day and down the next, if you run out of energy more than you used to, if you are tired of being tired, then perhaps it's time for you to change your thinking. Perhaps it's time to become skilled in creating your own abundance of energy. All you can lose is your chronic fatigue and your susceptibility to illness.

WE FORGET TO BE WELL

Most people talk about their state of health the way they do about the weather – as if they had no control over it. The implication is clear: they tolerate poor health, hoping sooner or later it that will go away. All they can do is resign themselves to whatever health or illness comes to them. Sadly, many surrender to this limitation whole-heartedly.

A friend went home for a holiday visit to her folks. During their conversation, her mother mentioned that a familiar neighbor, Mrs. Olson, was recently diagnosed as having cancer. The daughter immediately expressed shocked regret.

"Oh, well," the mother replied, " she is sixty years old."

Resignation to the imbalance of life's energy becomes the prime attitude of life for many people as they get older. Illness is considered normal and thus, inevitable. For some people it can also hold positive gains and other powerful meanings.

One day a friend broadcast to me with great gusto that his latest company physical examination indicated he had an ulcer.

"The doc says that I've got to eat special foods and ease off some with the work."

It was hard for me to believe, but his voice unmistakably sent another message: he was proud of himself! His next sentence confirmed it.

"Yep, I guess I'm just like the other bosses now!"

Apparently, the ulcer for this employee was a status symbol proving to his peers that he truly was a hard-working person. Like fatigue for a lot of other people, the ulcer was a badge of honor. With that attitude he will most likely hold on to his award and resist any thought of attaining optimal wellness.

People suffer not only from false resignation, lack of understanding, and misplaced sympathy about the life force, but from another, more debilitating ailment as well. There is an unsuspected malady that afflicts nearly everyone in our culture. It is like a slow-spreading, contagious plague. Professional advice does not help because professionals are likewise afflicted. This particular malady actually prepares people to become unwell in innumerable ways. It then keeps them unwell because it produces a subtle quality in their minds which undermines any awareness of its presence. Under its spell people deny that it has any bearing on their condition; it thrives invisibly. The malady is forgetfulness.

The malady is forgetfulness.

Under the sustained influence of energy-restricting habits – faulty nutrition, sporadic exercise, irregular breathing, fitful sleep, negative thinking, and chronic tiredness – we forget how well we are meant be. Our imbalanced lifestyle limits the amounts of energy we produce and use. We then restrict ourselves to minimal amounts, forgetting what it feels like to use more. Soon our forgetfulness confirms the state of mind that anything other than ebbing energy is quite impossible.

Exactly how do we get ourselves into this binding predicament? Quite simply, we do so by the way we mismanage the vitality of our lives. In our domestic and business decisions we arrange a lifestyle that insures the fever of forgetfulness. Our feelings, thoughts, and behavior towards ourselves and our environment support an idea of ourselves as a conglomerate of uncommunicative parts that have little to do with each other.

A Christian organization decided to include in their spiritual practices a demonstration of their sympathetic identity with the poor and starving peoples of the Third World. So they arranged with the local supermarket to purchase, at a greatly reduced price, the fruits and vegetables that would normally be thrown out. Sometimes the produce was so spoiled that the organization was not charged at all. They then began to practice Christian empathy with the poor by eating poor food. They hoped their frugality and charity would give a boost to their spiritual commitment. In a matter of days the majority of the community was sick in bed, suffering from fatigue, diarrhea, nausea, and headaches.

The group soon found alternative ways to identify with their brethren in the Third World, at last realizing the importance of healthy raw ingredients in their recipe for spiritual growth.

A young man in his early twenties came to me for help with his severe hay fever. His nostrils were totally closed, forcing him to breathe laboriously through his mouth. There was much sneezing and nose blowing, a constant headache, and red, running eyes. Over the years he had been to dozens of physicians and taken countless drugs for the problem. Nothing seemed to help.

It took ten minutes to teach him jal neti, the simple yogic nasal technique, used for centuries in many cultures around the world. After the last drop of water flowed out of his nose, he stood up, took a deep breath through his nostrils, and looked shocked.

"Wow! I feel just like when I was a kid on my skateboard. I haven't breathed like this since then. Why don't the doctors know about this?"

Simple, natural techniques, of course, are not given credence in our technological, pharmaceutical-controlled world. There is no money to be made in cleansing the nostrils; better to prescribe drugs and tell patients they'll have to "learn to live with it."

As I grew into my teens, I become a friend with a boy who lived across the street. We got into mischief together and spent a lot of time in each other's homes. The years went by and we both entered college – he to the local junior college, and I to the big, out-of-state university. I had never paid much attention to his father until I came home between semesters. The man seemed to be holding in immense anger and resentment whenever he saw me. He was very gruff to me, and criticized whatever I said or did. I wondered how he could find so much to criticize since I was not around much anymore. At first I paid little heed to his behavior, but as the years went on, visiting my friend became a chore whenever his father was there. One day I asked my friend what was wrong. He told me that when his father was a boy he won a scholarship to my university. At the last moment, his parents fell ill, forcing him to cancel college and take a low-paying job in the town factory. The man felt his lack of college had ruined his life, and he thought I did not demonstrate the gratitude, determination, and commitment appropriate for the priceless opportunity given to me.

No doubt the man had a point, but at what cost to his own well being? He was trapped in resentment and regret, rather than enjoying what he did have or doing something about the college degree he so desired.

Instead of caring for ourselves as a whole, we take a patchwork quilt approach to life. We load our minds with beliefs that curtail our future judgments about wellness. We ponder statistics that predict the various ills we are likely to incur. We give credence to the pseudo-physicians on television commercials who remind us of the need for frequent checkups, the necessity of taking our drugs, and the dangers of contemporary living. We turn an occasional ailment into the anxious standard through our fear. We think we have mindless bodies, akin to robots, repairable only by chemicals, surgery, or radiation. We believe professionals who tell us that personal attitudes and self-care are marginal to the promotion of our well being. We drive hard bargains for financial gain and postpone the importance of replenishing our energy. We struggle through our middle years as if we can disregard our bodies for the sake of financial success and a secure pension. We assume we can eat anything, anytime, since Rolaids are always near at hand. We see pain as a sign of hard work, accomplishment, and the need for repeated medication. We slowly wear out because we partition our bodies from our minds and our thoughts from our feelings. Our minds and bodies are like a couple who live together but seldom speak to each other, begrudging even the little they have in common. Our bodies and minds communicate only through rumor!

Because of this problem in intra-personal communication, our imbalanced lifestyle fosters susceptibility to disease: we set ourselves up for ill health.

....

"During my first year on the hospital wards, I was continually amazed by how little responsibility most patients took for their own health. About half the patients I saw that year had a preventable illness. Every time I saw a smoker with lung cancer or emphysema, a heavy drinker with liver disease, a fat, sedentary businessman with a heart attack ... I realized that medical care is not something to be left to doctors and other health workers."[3]

— Tom Ferguson, M.D.

....

Indeed, medication is the typical solution for all our problems. Whether the symptoms are mental, emotional, or physical, there are a host of drugs ready to be prescribed. While there are many life-saving drugs that have enabled people to live longer, pain-free lives, most commonly prescribed drugs are not only unnecessary, but also often harmful. Dr. Marc Lappe says that no antibiotics "can be said to have proven successful in truly eradicating any infectious disease in modern times."[4]

Treating the hundreds of symptoms of stress with drugs is particularly useless. The original problem usually remains unchanged; it is merely covered up. Often treating these ids-eases with drugs causes other diseases because the powerful 'curative' causes imbalance in the body's homeostasis. Prescription drugs are a poor choice, and one that invites diminishing returns:

1. Drugs do not eliminate the causes of illness.

2. Drugs engender new biological stresses.

3. Drugs undermine your confidence in your own self-reliance.

4. Drugs weaken your natural healing force.

It has been my observation that the customary administration of drugs produces dependency in patients. In fact, a co-dependency is usually established between physician and patient. Because they have been taught by family physicians, hospital emergencies, and media advertisements, people tend to seek recourse through drug prescriptions as their first line of coping with illness.

Enormous propaganda has been parlayed into building the illusion that miracle drugs are responsible for the decline of diseases and are the chief protector of the future.

R.R. Porter's study, for example, indicates that with improved
sanitation nearly 90 percent of the "total decline in death rate during
this epoch (1860–1965) had occurred prior to the introduction of
antibiotics."[6]

There is a curious parallel between farming and medicine. Farmers' reliance upon pesticides and herbicides is quite similar to the
medical profession's reliance upon drugs. Farmers are well aware
that healthy crops resist bugs and disease. Farmers have also learned
that pesticides make profit for chemical companies at the cost of
weakening the vitality of the land and creating a need for ever more
chemicals. In the 1930s, scientists noted seven species of bugs that
acquired resistance to pesticides. As the continual use of chemicals
for the soil increased, by 1984 there were at least 447 species that
were resistant.

It is no different for humans. The continual use of medical drugs
after World War II caused various bacteria in the human body to
mutate into more virulent strains, along with brand new inhabitants
that had never resided there before. In 1941 a physician would prescribe about 40,000 units of penicillin per day for four days as a cure
for pneumonia. In 1992, 24 million units per day were deployed with
no sign of patient recovery. Dr. Harold En states that bacteria that
cause infection are now "resistant to virtually all of the older antibiotics. The extensive use of antibiotics in the community and hospitals has fueled this crisis."[7] It seems we have yet to understand that
antibiotics, steroids, vaccinations, chemotherapy, and the pharmaceutical approach to health in general only camouflage the toxic devi-
talization of the life force, making us more susceptible to disease.

These observations are not isolated instances; they illustrate the
dominant medical protocol. Medicine's militant attempts to search
and destroy the "enemy bacteria and viruses" only provoke the body's
natural defenses to resist that much harder, sometimes in bizarre,

harmful ways. Thanks to medical drugs, previously harmless bacteria, such as E coli, have mutated into virulent forms that defy further medication. The prevalent notion that larger and more intense doses are the answer has failed abysmally. A possible glimmer of intelligent assessment appeared in 1990, when the Centers for Disease Control stated that the conventional drug treatment for gonorrhea should be abandoned because it was no longer working. Hope, however, soon faded. The new, replacement remedy was a more toxic and more expensive series of drugs.[8]

Medical practice does not seem to "get it." The tragic irony is that by relying upon drugs to kill disease, the physician instead increases the likelihood of repeat infections, as well as suppresses the very organic processes that keep health in good order – the immune system. Hans Selye, a pioneer in stress research, offers an important query:

....

"If a microbe is in or around us all the time and yet causes no disease until we are exposed to stress, what is the 'cause' of our illness, the microbe or the stress? ... In most instances the disease is due ... to the inadequacy of our reactions against the germ."[9]

....

Dr. Sheldon Cohen and his associates at Carnegie Mellon University also concluded that: "... stress is associated with the suppression of a general resistance process in the host, leaving persons susceptible to multiple infectious agents. Stress is associated with the suppression of many different immune processes, with similar results."[10]

Just as farmers and food-producing corporations are destroying healthy soil (which affects the food we eat) through unnecessary use of pesticides and herbicides, so too are physicians harming the health of their patients through the indiscriminate use of drugs. It seems to me that our "disease care system" has made scant use of the available knowledge of how to bolster the body and strengthen resistance to disease.

Should we therefore outlaw all medical drugs? Not at all. Just as chemical fertilizers can be advantageous to soil management, the careful dispensation of drugs can ameliorate disease and save lives in emergencies. The perplexing crisis for the medical community resides not in the sincere desire to benefit the patient, but in its mind-set devoted to chemical and surgical intervention. For the medical profession, the focus on pathology has evolved into a "pathological focus" upon the exclusive use of drugs for treatment. Perhaps the profession needs to be reminded of the words of Franz Ingelfinger, the former editor of the New England Journal of Medicine, who said that 85 percent of human illnesses are self-limiting, that is, within the reach of the person's innate healing resources.[11]

....

"The outright domination of intervention over self-reliance, in particular over psychophysiologic self-regulation, is not good for people or for society. It fosters dependence and represses human potential."[12]

– Dr. Elmer Green

....

Missing from the mentality of the medical establishment and the common understanding of patients is the recognition that the life force is trustworthy to work out its problems on its own when the natural requirements of the body and mind are adequately met. The mechanized aggression of modern medicine towards acute situations may be commendable in the emergency room, but the same approach fosters disasters in the treatment of chronic ailments. If we had a moratorium on hospital admittance, there would be a vast improvement in the general health of the country. People can make a difference in the state of their wellness by recognizing that palliatives like tranquilizers, flu shots, radiation, and headache pills jeopardize their future health.

ENERGY AT WILL

Given all these ideas about the energy of wellness and illness, what do you expect for your future? Do you want to sustain your current energy level? Would you want to have more energy? Would you like unlimited amounts of dynamism at your disposal? Do you want an energy that spreads throughout all the aspects of your being so that your body, emotions, imagination, thinking and intuition are integrated and strong? Do you want the energy to initiate a happier, healthier future?

Your present feelings of going downhill do not mean that you are losing the possibility for wellness, but only that you are forgetting how to get in touch with it. Rather than brood about your dwindling vitality, start to be concerned about your refusal to retrieve more of life's energy. Your procrastination is a sign that you are writing yourself off. Why do that?

Too often people endure energy loss for months, even years. They experience their vitality diminishing to lower and lower levels. They have forgotten how it feels to be vigorously well and consider the possibility of optimal wellness a fantasy, a joke. They appreciate their bodies less and less and they complain more and more. They then pay a terrible penalty: their negativity constricts their life force, preventing wellness and inviting disease. Inevitably they become philosophical about their plight: "Well, that's the way life goes."

Let's look at an example. Suppose you are getting tired and stiff – nothing serious, just annoying. Since the aches and fatigue do not impair you that much, you ignore them or perhaps take some recommended drugs. Soon, however, the feeling of fatigue becomes a steady companion. You wish it was otherwise but your work and your focus of attention becomes more and more disrupted by your weariness. You now begin to worry about the growing pain and fatigue as the quality of your work (and your emotions) suffers. You will then either go to a physician who will prescribe more drugs, or accept the fact that you are "falling apart" and learn to live with it.

Since this drama repeats itself quite often in our lives, let us analyze its three important features:

1. My feeling of tiredness

2. The state of my energy

3. How these two – tiredness and energy – are connected.

Can you feel energetic when you are tired? Hardly. When you are tired, you easily focus on your *feelings* of tiredness. Your tired condition exposes the poor status of your energy; you feel depleted.

On the other hand, when you are energetic you cannot focus on tiredness. Why not? Because you can *feel* only your level of energy. You do not feel tired because you sense high energy. You may remember the word "tired," you may recall that you felt like that often, but it is not the same as being tired. You are now in touch with an upgraded level of your life force.

The exchange between your feelings and the state of your energy is in constant communication. These two factors are differently but essentially connected because your feelings are part of the energy of your self-awareness, which is always in contact with your state of energy. Normally, your feelings about being either energetic or fatigued reflect the state of your energy.

The state of being tired, however, is meant to be temporary. Only when we ignore it does it become a problem. If our bodies get tired, it is difficult to think otherwise of anything else. We usually have to slow down or stop what we are doing and rest. Later, after nourishment, sleep, or some time to recuperate, we feel somewhat recharged. Typically, we think of rising each morning and "using up" our energy throughout the hours of the day until we come home tired from work. Then we relax through the evening and retire to sleep. If we allow our "tired" energy to become a pattern, we wake up nearly as tired as when we went to bed. After awhile, we assume that this is our norm. But we are tired because we identify with our fatigue; we *become* fatigued. We even say that in our language: I *am* tired.

Conversely, if we select our life force itself, rather than accede to temporary feelings, we *become* the life force and have it at our disposal. Thus when we feel tired, we immediately do something about it by engaging those resources that stimulate energy. We are reconnected immediately to our source of energy. Thus, we can disavow our negative feelings of fatigue and focus instead on choosing rejuvenation. Rejuvenation means that the energy patterns indicating tiredness reconstitute themselves into favorable patterns. So we transform the cycle of tiredness into a usable state of positive energy.

We reconstitute our energy by engaging the source of wellness. This innate process consists of more than the knowledge that the source exists; it involves communicating with it so that we can absorb and use its potential vitality. How do we do this? By consciously applying the skills of our six resources. As we have seen, the skills themselves lie within the broad horizon of life. Air, sunlight, water and space surround us; we breathe the vital air, the take in the vital sunlight through our skin and in our food. We walk briskly and rest. We relate with the community and revitalize ourselves in solitude. Life's energy awaits us when we know how to develop and harvest its potential. It is usable and renewable. It evades depletion unless we abuse it.

All events and activities take place upon the energy fields of life. How simple. Yet we overlook the fact that the basis for enjoying life is the balanced give and take of vitalizing energy constantly available within and about ourselves.

FINDING YOUR ROOTS

Have you ever noticed how little exercise is required for a muscle to improve its tone? The muscle is always ready and willing to improve its performance but, not knowing that, we usually convince ourselves that strengthening it would be too strenuous. Similarly, we neglect to take full advantage of the potential vitality inherent in our nature. It's always there; we simply do not see it. The awareness that we are deeply rooted in the life force is itself a resource always at hand.

You can easily change the quality of your life. The innate power of your life force provides the potential energy, your creative use of natural skills accesses it, and optimum wellness is the outcome. Your own skillful stimulation of your life force engenders its own vitality. Substantial changes in outlook and metabolism then occur. You feel better physically, emotionally, and mentally because you are increasing your vitality. More vitality means you feel and actually become stronger and healthier in body and mental outlook. Since your performance level develops in proportion to your sense of personal awareness, your increased vitality widens your recognition of life's abundant possibilities.

Adulthood is not an excuse for declining in wellness. If the rest of nature renews itself seasonally, why should human beings forego the opportunity? A tree readily absorbs and uses the abundant energy that the forest provides. It constantly renews itself, rooting itself more and more deeply into its potential vitality. Seasonal passages provide the environment for developing and growing, yet nature's bounty offers more than the tree can possibly absorb in any one season.

In like manner, your life force animates and organizes every cell in your body. Your body is renewable energy, an individualized expression of your life force. The bounty of life's resources – from the water you drink to the thoughts you think – always exceeds your grasp of them. At any moment, life's full potential is still to be elicited. A great privilege looms: to access, amplify, and renew life's energies in your self.

Contacting the life force demands a positive, willful intent on your part. This conscious choice immediately empowers your body and mind to make changes. Remember the last time you got really interested in the possibilities of an idea? Excitement flourished effortlessly; action rose spontaneously.

Likewise, the truth about you holds the imperishable potential of personal wellness. All you have to do is remind yourself that the energy for growth – physical, emotional, and mental – derives its momentum from the deliberate use of your natural resources. The conscious activation of each of your resources of attitude, breath, nutrition, movement, rest, and solitude, stimulates your life force. Coordinate these resources well and you have a force that transforms patterns of low energy into vitality.

In fact, you already call upon these same resources for getting through your day, but the crucial questions remain. How do you use these energy resources? Are they static or dynamic, homeostatically fixed or homeodynamically changeable? Do you overuse one while neglecting the other? Your use bodes ill or well for yourself; it impedes energy or facilitates vitality. You make the difference between a typical life and optimal wellness.

This quest for wellness is not a denial of illness and death, nor an obsessive desire to become the fittest aerobic agent on the block; rather, it is an invitation to examine your capacity for enjoying the energy of body and mind. That might not necessarily be perfect health, but it is an improved sense of well-being, whatever your bodily state. Optimal wellness is not immunity from risk or physical impairment any more than medical care is liberation from illness and death. Optimal wellness is the full use of our potential in order to realize the truth and significance of life.

How can we best organize our natural resources into self-care practices that promote optimal wellness? As we have seen, engendering wellness is the process of tapping the life force. It is a learned skill, an art.

....

Life force + creative skill = energy of wellness

....

By structuring our life force, we produce the energy outcomes that match our intent. The many forms of energy – gravity, magnetism, electricity – truly form part of the complexity of our nature, but our vital, conscious energy incorporates and uniquely unifies all of them. Wellness occurs when our life force is consciously and skillfully engaged.

ABUSE OF POWER

You have your bodily being because of the vital force pulsating in it. You feel emotions and think thoughts and run about only because of its dynamic presence. Place your hand on your wrist or over your heart and feel it pulsating through your body. There the equality ends, for each of us uses and abuses that power in a different way.

Abuse of life's energies takes many forms. Compare two of my friends. One is thirty-five, a successful, aggressive businessman. He is married, has an enviable income and no economic problems. Yet, getting a good night's sleep is rare for him. His commitment to building a prosperous life for his family and satisfying his own personal ambition leads him to deplete his energy. When he gets tired he pushes harder. His tired episodes are only problems to be fixed. He sees no gain without a lot of pain; he is the ideal over-achiever. His fatigue is starting to interfere with his sex life. He feels increasing vague pains during the day (which he resents), and "runs out of energy" on weekends (which he hides). He thinks success demands bullying his energy into compliance.

Another friend, fifty, has grown children. He has undergone several mild heart attacks, suffers digestive problems and stiff joints, medicates himself daily with five prescription drugs, and worries incessantly about how long he will be around to enjoy his pension. He broods on the thought of by-pass surgery but fears the possible complications. He jokingly remarks to his pitying spouse that he's mellowing. He feels more inclined to sit around the house, whine, and watch television than to get involved in tasks that require any sustained energy. He has a thousand excuses for not going fishing, his favorite hobby. He ponders the fitness program designed for people like himself down at the gym, a few blocks away. "It is too far to walk; besides it probably wouldn't do any good." Ironically, the numbing of the medication enforces his lassitude. When I visit him again next year I know he will repeat the same litany of complaints, only slower.

Neither man is ecstatic about his vitality, but without any immediate personal crisis, each is willing to tolerate the waning level of his life force. Their patterns of thinking and behavior towards themselves are consistent within the constraints of their chosen lifestyle. Uneven in their quotient of energy, they are, nevertheless, both progressing downhill to increasingly lower energy. They proclaim that no one, of course, enjoys perfect health.

In attempting to adapt to a situation that continually does not work well, one can analyze the recurring stress. It is very stressful when there is a disparity between the important demands in your life and your ability to facilitate them. Stress brings you to these unfamiliar limits of performance and, disturbing as it may be, it also serves a very good purpose: it gives you a chance to reexamine your ambition and/or your style of life. Your encounter with recurring stress means that it is time to revamp your approach within your current energy boundaries or else grow beyond them by enhancing your energy.

There are many ways to initiate a revision of your energy for handling recurring stress without arousing disequilibrium. An excellent method is a simple form of self-dialogue. In dialogue with your mind, you will discover that emotional energy can be monitored and reconstituted.

Once you have located the emotional stressor in your life, plan a time when you can calmly ponder it. Ask yourself some important questions:

Why does this affect me so much?
What is it that is REALLY upsetting me?

- DO NOT STRAIN for answers but simply allow your mind to survey the factors.

- CONVEY THEM to paper: the situation, the person(s), the time involved.

- FOCUS ON the specific feeling that always occurs to disturb you during the situation. Gently interrogate it.

- NOTE THE THOUGHTS that have feeling with them.

As you begin to experience some clarification of your stress, ask yourself two additional questions:

What is this confrontation revealing to me?

- STAY WITH THIS REVIEW, not to cast blame, but to examine the dynamics of the scenario, picking up spontaneous clues that arise because of your reflective state of mind. After some time your scrutiny will prompt other questions:

Why do I feel this way only under these circumstances?

Sometimes I can sense my stress coming on, so what is it in myself that is associated with the situation?

What can I change so it doesn't happen?

- GIVE YOUR MIND a chance to witness without arousing emotional intensity. This frees your mental energy from the constraints of the stress patterns so it can search amidst its vast experiences and learnings for the resolution. Sooner or later you will be able to move on to the next inquiry.

Once you have a sufficient sense of the cause of the stress, contemplate the second question: What way can I respond to this situation that will be advantageous to all parties?

🖋 INSTEAD OF JUSTIFYING your habitual response by reminding yourself of all the shortcomings on the other side, or grumbling the usual excuses, "It's his fault," "I can't change," "I deserve better," quietly examine the entire event for the purpose of changing your future.

🖋 ONCE THE ISSUE has been identified with sufficient clarity, your mind can energize your imagination for more choices. The energy of future choice is richer in its options than your history of response; the potential energy of your possible emotional patterns is broader than your customary judgment. How else could life proceed in these situations? It always evokes new choices from your intuitive consciousness.

Another method of expanding your own healing energy is personal research. It is your limited knowledge of yourself that restricts your self-assurance and your ability to change creatively. Personal research into your own life force and the quality of your life is rewarding. No academic degree is required for this research; just probing awareness.

Researching yourself is easy, accurate, and energizing. The only equipment required is your own body, mind, and spirit, a sense of curiosity, and the natural creative tools, which you already possess. You come fully equipped; your only investment is time. Just as it takes time to become unwell, so does it take time to become well. The research is carried out by performing the experiments following each chapter in this book and observing what happens to your energy. You observe yourself stimulate an energy change in yourself. You are the experiment, and you are the experimenter.

There is a profound difference between *performing* and *being* a laboratory experiment. Laboratory results are external to the scientist; she or he dispatches them to laboratory charts and reports. When you *are* the laboratory, your energy results reside in you. The scientist is exhilarated by graphic results; you are exhilarated by the infusion of wellness energy. When you experiment with the self-care practices in this book, you will learn that research on the self renews the researcher.

Performing self-research also involves you in a rewarding conspiracy with the various energy fields of life. Your mind monitors its own energy as it goes about its business of fulfilling its desires, provided you pay attention. This experience of conscious feedback allows you to direct and measure the energy force of your resources. Like a servo device, you make adjustments as you proceed, modifying the interaction of mind and body in accordance with the changing environment, even upgrading its vitality. The upgrading requires time. A new habit must be born, then established for stability and reliability. The mental and biological changes that occur are activated not only to bring you back to homeostasis but also to sponsor new metabolic exchanges, voluntarily created within your whole energy field and experienced as an increase in energy. With the new habit a new awareness emerges in your field of perception and a new ability to execute behavior better. Homeostasis now takes it cue from homeodynamics – actualizing the potential for positive change in the entire complex of your energy field.

....

"In a physiological sense, we could not survive without homeostasis, but it is important to know that continuous pressure can modify homeostatic balance. Homeostasis keeps us healthy and bouncing back from the strains and stresses of life – up to a point. If we are continuously reacting to stress, then homeostatic balances gradually shift, for they are not permanently fixed, and the undesirable result in our bodies is called psychosomatic disease. If such a disease does develop, then homeostasis actively maintains it until we do something about it."[3]

– Elmer and Alyce Green

....

These profound changes are created, as well as impeded, because the life force functions at various levels within its own mind-body energy field. The experience of chronic stress, for example, has a restrictive influence upon the psychosomatic energy field, causing dysfunctional patterns of energy performance that are evident in your behavior. Homeostasis undergoes trauma which produces a pervasive and often non-specific impact upon the entire human organism and results in an unpredictable range of symptoms from vague weariness with life to sporadic chest pains to sudden headaches, anxiety, and impotence.

Wellness is nearby when rigid unconscious patterns of energy are re-synthesized into newer, richer, flexible ones. This body-mind transformation occurs when sufficient stimulation of the life force reorganizes its energy patterns. One is then able to understand the self in new ways and gain some beneficial extension on the future.

Thus, you can express your capacities for living in accordance with the experience of your own changed energy. Even when there is no presence of obvious pathology, the proper combination of your self-regulated resources will expand your current limits of homeostasis, raising your level of self-approval and perceptual performance. The quality of your lifestyle advances.

INTEGRATING YOUR ENERGY

As this book has said in many ways, life's resources become progressively more usable as one implements them. Your sense of bodily awareness grows keener, for example, with careful breathing, or movement, or rest, enabling you to be less susceptible to unconscious stress. Anxious fear of pain and disease wanes. It's a no-fuss, no-expense procedure. Awareness replaces amnesia. Ample energy inspires new self-confidence. Your experiments on yourself bring the power of their energy to your awareness. You have wandered into the grove of possibilities. The trees are ripe. What will you choose to do – erect fences or pluck fruit?

Experimenting with your six resources of attitude, breath, diet, movement, rest, solitude changes your understanding about your personal biology. Instead of judging yourself as a tiring, aging machine, you will regard yourself as a quickening life force. From this viewpoint, your body and mind constitute an individualized field of energy capable of producing self-directed change for the stages of wellness. Like a living tree, your assimilation of energy as sunlight, food, water, air, and movement charges you with more energy. You absorb energy from the environment and you exude energy into the environment. You understand that your cells are vital aggregates of corpuscular energy, your bodily fluids are flowing energy, your bones are calcareous energy, your skin is fibrous energy, your senses are energy receivers, your thoughts are energy forms extending through the field of your body. Walking, running, or sitting, your body constantly emits the energy of heat and vapor.

The solid matter of your body is condensed energy; your mind with its thoughts and feelings is finer energy. You are not a body plus mind plus energy but embodied/mentalized energy, differentiated and organized into a single, living whole. Your body is a flexible mass of energy amenable to the vibration of your thought forms. Your person is a congregation of varying, systemic patterns of energy, subject to energy exchanges with your environment as well as with your own energy of thoughts and feelings.

> Listening to your heartbeat, you hear its muscular discharge of energy.
> Taking your pulse, you feel the rhythmic energy of the blood's motion.
> Watching your breathing, you sense the lungs' energy of expansion and contraction.
> Walking briskly, you use the energy of locomotion.
> Emoting, you experience the sensual force of your energy.
> Worrying, you feel the depletion of your energy.
> Stressed, you sense the constriction of your energy.
> Enjoying sex, you share your energy intimately with another.
> Playing, you know the pleasure of your energy.
> Meditating, you know the peace and freedom of your energy.

Because you are a dynamic individuation of living, self-renewing energy, your continuing work with your six resources permits you to compose, alter, modify, strengthen, and expand your energy to grow, to heal, and to forestall the aging process. Change is an essential dimension of your being in time and space. The pursuit of optimal wellness gives you the leverage to make the changes on your own terms.

MOVING INTO LIFE

Each of us carries the potential to die as well as to live. Why hurry the former? Why limit yourself to increasing illness because statistics and your neighbors say you should? The slightest tendency toward some aspect of wellness can multiply change throughout your entire person. Whatever your deficits, the closer you get to life's resources the stronger your vitality becomes.

A paraplegic painting with a brush held between his teeth exudes more force of life than a successful entrepreneur contemplating his third coronary bypass. The innate purpose of energy is to constantly reorganize itself in order for you to benefit from life's abundance. When you consider your body as the materialization of your life force, you have the leverage to change it much more readily than someone who presumes a static division between mind and body. If you feel you must wear out, why not wear out as a unit, body and mind together? If we deny an attitude of wholeness, we move closer to pain. We heal and grow when we see ourselves as fully integrated beings.

The advantage of this perspective is that it allows a conceptual approach to living that does not get in its own way. It's not just a mind trip. Do you recall playing vigorous games outdoors with your friends? Remember all the energy you exerted? Afterwards, you may have been winded and bruised, but you were nonetheless permanently enriched by the activity. Your future was enhanced. Whether your life force converts raw vegetables into edible food or restores your depleted energy through a good night's sleep or a few hours alone, you can learn how to use the energy changes for your personal wellness. You can make a qualitative and quantitative difference in your energy. That difference can be integrated, resorted to again and again and, when depleted, renewed. Once you initiate your experiments, you will know that your life force is never utterly bound nor irretrievably restricted by the energy patterns of your past. You can reset the limitations of your energy – you can choose its future. Without executing your choice, however, your experience of life remains the same. A host of experiences await your use but you will miss them. You miss experiencing the process of acting it out, you miss experiencing the completion, and you miss experiencing the new possibilities along the way.

You can contact your life force and use its power or you can decline the invitation. Your decision, however, forms your attitude to life and your future wellness.

PRACTICE SESSION

Visualization Exercise

Visualization is a very helpful and powerful technique. It may be difficult for some people until it is combined with relaxation. It is harder to hold an image than a thought. With practice, however, you can learn to steady your imagination and allow your body-mind complex to experience the benefits of visualization. Visualizing can easily reduce your tension as well as open your creative intuition.

Here is a visualization practice for releasing residual tension.

- LIE DOWN on your back on a firm surface. Place a small pillow under your head. Breathe diaphragmatically for a few minutes, and then do the practice of progressive relaxation.

- WHEN YOU HAVE COMPLETED progressive relaxation, imagine your inhalation as waves of warm, energizing vitality entering your body. Imagine your exhalation as departing waves of energy. You can also 'feel' the moving energy as it travels through your body.

- NOW VISUALIZE a scene that promotes the feeling you wish – a place that helps you feel calm, happy, peaceful. It might be the seashore where you watch the ebb and flow of the waves. It might be a hill where you watch the fluffy, white clouds slowly floating by in a vast, blue sky. It might be a forest where you watch towering pine trees gently moving their branches in the wind.

- KEEP WATCHING the scene as you breathe calmly, slowly, and evenly. Continue this visualization for five to fifteen minutes, and then gently open your eyes.

CHAPTER 9

Recreating Yourself

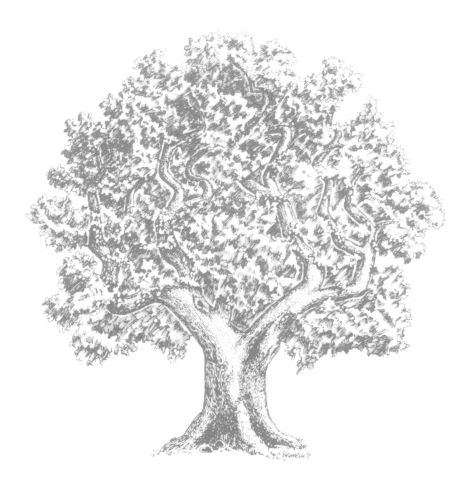

A MAN ONCE REMARKED that he had a terrific advantage over others when he was a teenager – he suffered from polio. He had the use of his hearing and slight speech, but the only part of his body he could move was his eyes. Lying in bed he pondered, above all things, how he could entertain himself. So he decided to observe his family.

Soon he discovered the nonverbal body language of his loved ones. A whole new learning horizon opened to him. He especially studied his baby sister. Intensely watching her creep, slip, and struggle to stand up, he painstakingly relearned the complicated dynamics involved for that task.

One afternoon his parents strapped him into his rocking chair as usual, and then left the room. As he thought about wanting to look out the window many feet away, the rocker swayed slightly. Surprised, he began to experiment with his will and its possible communication with his unmovable body. Somehow he was able to rock the chair to the window!

His mind refused to accept the verdict of paralysis that was given to his body. Thus began years of self-research into the incredible power of intent, learning new ways to use his innate energy. He honed his power of observation to profound levels and realized the total communication between intent of the mind and acquiescence of the body. Eventually he achieved physical rehabilitation. This man was Milton Erickson, a pioneer in mind-body communication and one of America's foremost counselors. By entertaining himself with learning, he altered his patterns of energy. By provoking his life force, he transformed the routine knowledge of his handicap into an opportunity for profound growth in self-awareness and universal therapy. He became a genius in fostering self-healing.

CREATIVITY AND WELLNESS

The program of The Wellness Tree starts from the conviction that you are a holistic being – an intelligent, organic, living energy field which can improve, rehabilitate, and increase your living energy on call. When we choose progressive amnesia, we steadily forget the truth of the living interplay of energy among our feelings, images, thoughts, body, behavior, and environment. As Dr. Erickson proved, the mind has vast stores of creative potential, waiting to be tapped for our personal and community benefit. As with other human potentials, creativity must be acknowledged and accepted in order to be made actual.

You have heard the word "creativity" used in many different ways. Artistic and business circles compete with the word, the advertising world plans creative ads, authors write creative books, there are creative cooking and creative decorating classes, there is even creative financing for your purchases. When we speak of creativity for wellness, however, we propose a different meaning:

....

Creativity is the power to induce vitality.

....

When you use your creativity for wellness, you apply wholly natural skills to yourself in order to induce new vitality. You not only restore yourself: you create rejuvenation, bringing into existence that which was not there before. Creativity is closely related to the six resources we have been studying. The feeling you evoke as you use them spontaneously increases the awareness of your vital force. With growing awareness you are reminded that you can call forth the needed energy again and again. Your metabolism improves; you feel more vitality because you are more alive. Since you consciously choose to invigorate yourself, your increased vitality expands your awareness of that vitality. Because the self-care skills root you deeply into the energy of your life force, your body and mind improve their communication, and open the door to intuitive creativity.

In searching for the tree of life within yourself, you may recall that a tree in the forest succeeds itself through its seeds. Its fruit contains the seeds of survival and re-creation. By learning intuitive creativity you can discover the "seeds" of your creative consciousness, which not only germinate survival but also hold the embryo of change that guarantees an optimum future. You draw upon a vast, natural, hidden force that guides the re-creation of your physiological processes as well as inspiring new possibilities for living.

MEDIUM FOR CHANGE

In order to grasp the possibilities of intuitive creativity, let us compare it with the experience of watching a film. At the cinema, a story unfolds on the screen before you. As your mind follows the story, you respond emotionally. The more you are involved in the film, the more and varied are your feelings. Time flies by unnoticed when the story intrigues you. If a physician were attending you, he would detect changes in your pulse rate, heart beat, breath rate, blood pressure, and the contraction or release of muscles. These bodily changes are consistent with the emotions stimulated by your attention to the film. Not only does your mood change in reference to the story; your whole person responds to it.

All of this experience is primarily taking place through the medium of images. The combination of sound and sight supply your imagination with those sense impressions that allow you to think and feel the way you do. You are not a detached onlooker but an emotional participant in the scenes alternating upon the screen. You empathize, you contribute your active attention.

We might also consider the moving images of the film to be fixtures. You did not fabricate them. They do not alter in any way with continual showings. If they are not to your liking, there is nothing you can do about them. Over a period of time, however, if you see the movie again and again, you can easily change your original emotional response. That first flush can dwindle, increase, or utterly vanish, and so can your bodily responses. The point we are making here is that the cinema is pretense. In viewing a film we are pretending reality. The scenes depicted upon the screen are not real; they are mechanical images so ingeniously contrived as to typify the real. We enter into active participation with the screen through our imagination, and for awhile we construe the moving images as part of our life. As long as we accept the pretense we respond appropriately, which means we elicit cognitive, emotional, and bodily changes in ourselves in direct reference to the film images.

This discussion demonstrates an important relationship, namely, the relationship between your mental images and your body. Imagination stimulates bodily behavior. As long as there is some attention paid to the screen images, there is a definite emotional response on your part. You might recall sharing a film with a friend, and each of you being provoked to different responses.

Intensity of response, however, is another matter. Some people who enjoy *Gone With the Wind* with its images of romance and heroics against a rich, historical background, may be somewhat bored with the futuristic *Star Wars*. While many people can appreciate and talk about the same images, the special feeling they have for them assumes a personal contribution on the viewer's part. The tension between Rhett Butler and Scarlet O'Hara holds a certain fascination for some people that others cannot appreciate. Same image, different response. Likewise, an old letter, photograph, or household item, quite minor in itself, may hold riches of emotion for its possessor. Equally so, the imaging of past experiences in our mind can evoke an intensity of emotional depth that nothing current in that person's life can emulate.

Meaning influences our emotional response.

In this way, images can bear a symbolic value for us that may not be apparent nor anticipated by someone else. An invitation to a boat ride on the lake may evoke a storm of tension in someone who cannot swim, and suffered a near drowning episode in childhood. To a fisherman reminiscing over his favorite pastime, the invitation evokes other emotions. Meaning influences our emotional response. We do not respond to an image because it's an image; we respond for the significance it possesses for us.

AN EXPERIMENT IN TIME REVERSAL

Some years ago, Professor Ellen Langer of Harvard University sent out an intriguing invitation to elderly men in the Boston area. She invited a number of 75- to 85-year-old men to a luxurious, secluded building in rural New England for a weeklong retreat. The chosen men were divided into two groups and instructed as to their duties.

Group A entered a building which was transformed to vintage 1959, more than twenty years earlier. Furniture, radio music, magazines and books, food packages, clothing, and decoration were all implements used in the 50's. Movies and recordings of people famous in that era were provided. As they donned the old clothes and sat in the old furniture, they were instructed to imagine themselves once again in 1959. All conversations were restricted to talk of 1959 or earlier, but they were to speak and act and think as if they were actually once again in 1959. They were to generate the ideas, feelings, and actions that belonged to them in the fifties. They were to help engage each other in reliving their lives.

Group B entered a normal building for their five-day retreat. They were instructed to continue living as they usually did, but to reminisce often about 1959 and their lives in the fifties. They were encouraged to assist each other in reminiscing about the past.

Before, during, and after the experiment physical and psychological tests were make of all the subjects. The results were astounding. The men in Group A showed drastic bodily and mental changes: their fingers lengthened and regained joint flexibility, they carried themselves more erect while sitting and standing, they walked with a spring in their step, their hearing and sight become keener, hand strength increased, memory improved, response to recognition tests was quicker and more accurate than before, and overall performance on intelligence tests was improved. Photos of Group A after the retreat showed men who looked at least three years younger than a week earlier.

Group B had no such results. For the most part, all the measured abilities remained the same as when they entered the retreat except that joint flexibility decreased for one-third of the men, response to recognition tests was slower than the other group, and overall performance on intelligence tests declined for one-fourth of the men.[1]

This experiment shows the power of creative imagination. It also shows that the decrements of aging are not as fixed as we would assume. Aging, like stress and time, is an inner evaluation about the world around us, and thus its ravages may be just as malleable as our beliefs about our future. For the men who had a postcard visit of the past from the comfort of the present, history was irreversible. Contemplating the past without an emotional commitment leaves it an abstraction. It is the full-bodied visit to the past that enables one to reconstruct the present. For those who dissolved their beliefs and their years into the energy of a happier time, history was re-created, as were they themselves.

Reframing energy in this way is one of the creative tools available to us when we are aware of our innate power. Milton Erickson discovered that time-bound memories are revisable. Through pioneering hypnotic trances in time reversal, he enabled his clients to reframe their lives to the future without being impeded with the baggage of the past. Perhaps we are all suffering from premature aging, but time, body rigidity, emotional pain and mental conditioning can all come under conscious direction. The experimenters in the study above intentionally collapsed their historic past into their current present and reaped the benefits of that energizing. Their conscious and unconscious collaborated in realigning themselves. If unprepared citizens could demonstrate such deconditioning, what could be done by those who are aware of the power of wellness?

....

On Winston Churchill's eighty-second birthday, a young photographer told him, "I hope I may have the privilege of taking your picture again when you are 100." Churchill replied, "No reason why you shouldn't if you continue to look after your health."

....

THE MIND AS CINEMA

Artists do not need scientific evidence to know that the power of the imagination is unlimited, but you might need to be convinced of the power of your own imagination. With the practice of intuitive creativity a whole new vista opens before you – a vista by which you can explore the inner terrain of your intuitive consciousness for its healing benefits.

In 1908 Dr. Edmund Jacobson, one of the early explorers of relaxation techniques for clinical use, presented abundant evidence to show the interdependence of mind and muscles. In his experiments, the subjects imagined using a particular muscle while not actually doing so. The act of imagination alone produced measurable bursts of muscle activity.[2]

From decades of experiments, evidence shows that while people believed anxiety and tension were caused by their outer circumstances, it was actually the pattern of images in their minds that produced muscle tension in their bodies. Our muscular responses to our experiences are retained as energy patterns in our memory. Thus, when we mentally review a situation – actual or pretense – those image patterns in our memory reactivate the stress pattern in our body. Some of these imagery patterns are so rigid that they affect our physical posture. When we are stressed, we show the strain in our facial muscles, our speech, our sleep, our eating habits, the sound of our voice, our gait. Worry gets into our tissues. We are so preoccupied with meeting life's tasks that we are hardly aware of the sustained tension in our bodies except when it becomes acutely painful.

We must not underestimate how much our images, especially images of ourselves, influences our moods, the direction of our lives, the solving of our problems. Of course, if we have never spent time experimenting with mental images, then it is hard to believe that we could make much difference in every area of our lives. Most of the time we rely upon an outside source to affect our disposition. When we need a mood change, we go outside to find it. We go to a sport event, we go to a restaurant, and we take a walk in the park or around the block. Hence, we presume that our thoughts, feelings, and images about ourselves are more insinuated by the environment and outer circumstances than by the resources within ourselves. It seems almost unnatural to propose that we could alter or devise our inner environment and thus increase our freedom to choose a mood or change our body and experience life anew.

Nevertheless, the process of intuitive creativity opposes the assumption that the way we feel about ourselves is necessarily determined by the occurrences around us and, especially, by our personal history. There is no doubt that the outer world provides us with our information about life. But what we do with the information, how to appreciate, evaluate, and respond to it, is one of two crucial factors in promoting the way we feel. The other factor is our ability to invoke the energy of our creative consciousness and elicit its dynamics.

The intimate, complex relationships between imagination, body, and mental images that influence your bodily functions provide a biological and psychological basis for the experience of intuitive creativity. We are able choose a process of conscious relaxation to engender a particular inner environment. Then, from the wellsprings of that environment appropriate images arise for changing the direction and behavior of our energy in accordance with our plans. The result is not arbitrary. With practice, anyone can learn to evoke desired images and use them for initiating preferred change. At the same time, it is quite possible to reverse habituated image patterns that are wasting energy and interfering with personal progress.

In this regard, the practice of intuitive creativity differs from meditation. In meditation, the goal is to proceed beyond thought and image, entering creative consciousness and proceeding further into stillness. The information generated in meditation does not arise merely as an intellectual concept; it is the natural occupation of the discursive level of consciousness. Intuitive creativity generates symbolic images, even a complex vision that can summarize the very resolution that you seek. Gaining access to this level of awareness is not strictly a thinking process, yet it entails a series of cognitive steps which involves the entire complex of body, breath, emotions, and relaxed attention. Intuitive creativity enters the creative consciousness and there solicits information for practical use.

IMAGINATION CONSTRUCTS CHANGE

Read the following experiment and then try it for yourself:

Sit erect.
Gently close your eyes.
Settle down for a few minutes by breathing diaphragmatically.
See in your mind an opened white umbrella with blue polka dots.

Now see the dots as yellow.
Now see them red.
Now see them yellow and red.
Turn them back to blue.
Now alternately shrink and enlarge the umbrella.
Close the umbrella.
Open your eyes.

During this deliberate imagining, it may have been hard to hold the object steady and the colors crisply. Certain objects are easier to hold than others are, but with practice you can improve the duration and the clarity of the images.

After reading the following, try this other experiment:

Sit erect.
Close your eyes.
Settle down with diaphragmatic breathing for about two minutes.
Select a pleasant location for your next vacation.
Compose in detail all the attractive aspects found there.
Just allow the images to develop on their own.
Dwell upon those images for awhile.
Now make them brighter, stronger.
Note your accompanying feelings.
Open your eyes.

These two simple experiments introduce us to an inner world. They also raise some intriguing questions. From where do I get the energy of imaging? How far can I imagine number, size, figure, color, and motion? Which image evokes the greatest response in me?

We can construct and retrieve past episodes in whole or part – like the umbrella scene – and review them or remake them. We can borrow from the vast library of images in our memory and compose something entirely new in our imagination. We can feel the effect of these images in the energy of our mind and body. It does not matter if the images are still or moving, for we can propose, in fairy-tale fashion, unorthodox images: trees that talk, flowers that sing, animals that behave like people. We have that power in our imagination. In fact, without the imagination of the listeners, a storyteller, a legend maker, would be out of a job.

As we become more familiar with the power of our imagination, it becomes quite apparent that it is truly an unbounded terrain, an inner form of outer space, existing for our exploration. In addition to composing images, we can search into the imagination and find all sorts of images, complete or fragmented, already composed. The emotional import of their value can, should we so desire, change our feelings from day to day. Reliving the past is a common experience, but the possibilities of remaking the present through imaging, and projecting the future as precisely as one wishes, may come as a surprise.

Using your imagination for promoting salutary change is a matter of simple practice. For that purpose, familiarize yourself with two different approaches to active imaging. In the first way, you compose your image and focus on it with concentrated ease. The concentration should not be forceful or tense like a muscle contraction, but more akin to a quiet gaze from a hilltop. It involves no harsh determination. Moving or static, abstract or concrete, an event or a scene, use whatever images you think appropriate for your prescribed goal. Do not force your attention but merely allow your feelings to respond appropriately to the image.

The second approach involves a vigorous composition of images in which you dramatize, often in symbolic style, the process you desire to occur. Thus you could choose aggressive, even violent, scenes where you or your representative emerges the victor in a struggle, or a series of adventurous encounters representing the triumph of your positive goal. Your calm exterior belies the stimulating engagement of your inner attention. This technique can also be used for improving any skill for the marketplace or for personal relations. It can be used for improving body coordination by visualizing the event – tennis, track, swimming, dancing, etc. – in the exact sequence you wish to perform it. Athletes are beginning to appreciate the power of such imaging for improving their sport. Within your imagination you simply detail the flow of the event.

The only restriction for the imagination seems to be the ingenuity of the image maker. On the field of your imagination, you become your own scriptwriter, producer, director, viewer and critic. In choosing either the first or second method, it is important that you remind yourself that you are in charge; you orchestrate the images and savor the process.

One day a retired British army officer came to me for help with his recurring nightmares. He had endured incarceration in a Japanese POW camp for nearly four years during World War II. His duty had been to help build the famous bridge over the river Kwai. In recent years, memories of this horrendous episode afflicted him at night, making him relive all the torture. Once again he felt powerless before his adversaries. Once again he endured the exhausting work. He would wake with stiffness throughout his body and a great reluctance to venture outdoors.

He learned the practice of progressive relaxation, and discovered that by actively imaging himself back in my office doing the practice, the gripping fear of his nightmare slackened. By using the office image, he reconstructed his emotional energy and gave his memory a new, powerful, positive experience to relive. He progressed until he finally distanced himself from the war memories, and gradually disassociated himself from them completely. He brought his energy under control and soon slept without incident.

The creative power of the mind often sustains memories that require recontextualizing in order to integrate that energy into ways we want it to go. The energy of any inner conflicts that arise can be changed through the power of imagination. The outcome is obvious: fewer hassles from within and an improvement in overall wellness.

CONTACTING CREATIVE CONSCIOUSNESS

The previous descriptions have explored the immediate dynamics of rational imagery that are available to the mind at its ordinary consciousness. There is yet another dimension to the power of images that brings the practitioner to a vast region of creative awareness. Creative consciousness is a much subtler area of awareness although it is not always easy to attain. Sometimes it asserts itself spontaneously. Many people recall incidents of long, frustrated sieges of effort to resolve a problem only to watch their rational efforts fail. Then suddenly the unexpected solution occurred to them, apparently out of nowhere.

Such was the case with a nineteenth-century German chemist, Friedrich Kekule von Stradonitz, who had a series of reveries:

One fine, summer evening I was returning by the last omnibus, "outside" as usual, through the deserted streets of the metropolis ... I fell into a reverie, and lo! the atoms were gamboling before my eyes.... I saw how, frequently, two smaller atoms united to form a pair, how a larger one embraced two smaller ones ... I saw how the larger ones formed a chain. I spent part of the night putting on paper the sketches of these dream forms.

The last 'dreams' in this series led von Stradonitz to a brilliant discovery in organic chemistry. He realized that some organic compounds exist, surprisingly, in closed rings:

I turned my chair to the fire and dozed. Again the atoms were gamboling before my eyes ... long rows, sometimes more closely fitted together, all turning and twisting in snakelike motion. But look! What was that? One of the snakes had seized hold of its own tail, and the form whirled mockingly before my eyes. As if by a flash of lightening I awoke ...[3]

While many such insights are sudden breakthroughs, the energy of creativity can also be enticed to perform. As we learn from Kekule, contacting your creative consciousness is similar to dozing, like being on the verge of sleep. But entering the level of creative awareness can also be a planned reverie. Until you are familiar with your mind's dynamics, keeping calm and aware takes skillful concentration. In journeying inward to this creative region, you must relinquish any pre-planned composition of images, although they show up spontaneously along the way. You simply create those inner, comfortable conditions that permit the life force to respond in its own way to your intent.

During your quieting, an energy shift occurs from left hemispheric brain dominance to right, or to an even balance of both. Accompanying this shift, peripheral warmth increases in the body. This is associated with a sense of heaviness or, in some instances, lightness. It is not uncommon for some people to arrive in this state within ten minutes, while for others it may take many days of practice to attain this creative condition.

When you are relaxed and comfortable, make your request for an answer to the problem or question you have. Refrain from actively composing any images. Instead keep yourself in an alert, receptive state of waiting so that your creative consciousness can communicate its images in reply. The answer may come in a variety of ways. You may experience various types of images – some visual, some kinesthetic (feeling), and some auricular (sound). As in the state of meditation, you witness the information. It may take the form of symbols, concepts, feelings, and geometric patterns – favorable or unfavorable. Entire stories may unfold or merely pieces of a larger puzzle. When the information surfaces, the steady state of your mood allows you to inspect it without provoking an emotional reaction. Afterwards you may need to interpret some of the information.

Besides receiving answers to problems, there are at least two other uses for this state of intuitive communication. You can reprogram your body in very specific ways and you can project plans for your future behavior. In order to do this, once again, attain a quiet, comfortable state of mind. Then imagine the changes in behavior, mood, energy levels or body systems that you desire. You choose the image and play out the scenario. You may, for example, heal a cut or sprain by seeing the area totally healed. Some people will visualize a scene; others will give a clear command with no elaboration.

In either case, you simply install the desire upon the screen of the creative consciousness and let it be. At that moment, your unconscious is like a genie, ready to do your bidding. Close out the session by acknowledging to yourself that the work has been assigned. Do not tamper with it. A good gardener does not dig up his seeds for inspection after they are carefully planted, so like a gardener, allow your recreation to continue on its own. Trust your unconscious. Then gently and slowly come back to ordinary awareness.

The second use repeats these steps but actively implements those images concerned with your future accomplishments. For example, you might wish to increase your public speaking skills by composing a scene of yourself successfully delivering a speech to an appreciative audience. Allow these images to be sensually composed in their appropriate setting. Make sure that the images of your future desires generate the appropriate emotions. You must be imaginatively involved with the experience in body and mind as it unfolds in order to stimulate your unconscious participation.

Entry into the creative sphere of consciousness is a self-learned and self-regulated skill. When using it for optimal wellness, there are two important implications. First, the gradual familiarity with the unexplored regions of your mind allows you to solicit clues and information about your body and your behavior that normally exceeds the reach of discursive awareness, but which can be quite useful. Additional unplanned bonuses can also emerge; you could gain personal insight, see things in a different context, or spot a new connection between ideas.

Second, the familiarity with the level of creative perception fosters self-awareness of both your psychological and physiological processes. You become aware of vital information about yourself which inspires control and direction over your bodily and rational energy. In terms of the biology of consciousness, you learn that your brain's limbic system – the home of emotions – and the viscera are intimately connected.

You can train your intuition. It is not a random, hit or miss venture but a systematic process guided by intent. It is as if you were supervising conference calls between various levels of consciousness; you eavesdrop on otherwise hidden, subliminal territory – your brain's theta state. Your ability to interrogate the wellsprings of creativity, elicit replies, project commands for your future, and reprogram your biological stresses becomes operative once you accept its possibility. The images you use for promoting vital change are not mere suggestions; they reconstitute your energy, inducing a new synthesis of your experiential life.

Your creative consciousness already knows how to heal; it also knows how to implement what is best for your talents, real and potential. Consequently, when you arrange the proper conditions, the renewing power of your life force evokes new patterns of conscious information which you can draw upon.

When you begin the exercise in creative consciousness, lie down on a firm, comfortable surface or sit in a comfortable chair. Close your eyes and lips gently. Breathe diaphragmatically and focus your attention inwardly as in meditation. Maintain diaphragmatic breathing throughout the imaging experience.

There are four factors that quicken creativity in the exercise:

1. Intend. Decide in advance the effect or change you want to achieve. Random attempts usually fail. Approach the creative consciousness seriously and without anxiety.

2. Prime. Entering creative consciousness is comparable to the practice of meditation; it requires a restful condition. Progressive relaxation induces the kind of inner feeling of comfort and the release of tension that is a prelude for reaching this subtle level of awareness.

3. Compose. If you choose to image changes by deliberate composition, then shape images that are consistent with your intent. For example, if you want to increase the temperature of your cold hands then do not visualize yourself in a winter climate. Spontaneous images will arise; you decide whether they fit with your instructions. If you are consulting your creative consciousness with a request then wait in silence for its message, remembering that the message could be information that you need rather than want.

4. Dwell. When you install the appropriate images, simply breathe slowly and allow your attention to remain with them. You are creating an energy form in your mind that symbolizes your intention. Do not analyze the scene as it occurs. Instead, stay in a learning mood; be present with it in all its sensual details. Allow yourself to dwell approvingly upon the scene. Your mind may flit here and there, parts of the scene may vanish, but continue anyway. Do not be too concerned with distractions. After you sense satisfaction, bring the process to closure in a relaxed way.

DESIGN FOR WELLNESS

When you assume conscious responsibility for your life forces, and for your wellness, you are in the business of "styling" your energy. You make it do what you want. Instead of waiting for your next droop of energy, for example, you can stop the depletion scenario by concentrating on stimulating your vitality. The creation of an optimal lifestyle does not mean incorporating quantities of new things to worry about; instead, you energize a lifestyle that is no longer susceptible to chronic wear and tear. You do not complicate your life, you simply change its energy flow. You "style" your energy, you design it to fit your needs and meet your goals through the application of your creative skills. When you execute them with a conscious intent, you reorganize your energy flow, enabling the life force to optimize your vitality. You then move into a new physical future by amplifying your life force.

Life's secrets are so obvious. Think back to the time when you pondered a change in your routine. Walking to work, getting up earlier, a different diet, attending a workshop, a course in writing, music, painting, computers, contact bridge, whatever. You started with a slight revision of your lifestyle. From awkward and uncomfortable beginnings, you gradually got control over what you were doing. You may not have become an expert, but your practice changed you. Some development occurred in you and you felt it. The external help you may have received does not account for your change; all the coaching in the world is impotent unless you decide and act on it. However clumsy you may have felt about yourself, the result of your practice was improvement, and you knew that further improvement lay in the future. What actually happened? You went from a condition of indifferent potential energy to a condition of organized energy. You increased your power to live.

A few questions are in order. Where did the power to make the change reside? How was the power to make the change implemented? The answer to both questions is *you*. The power came from your innate resources – your mind, your time and effort, your body. It does not matter how long your effort endured or how incomplete your outcome. The point is, you empowered the change.

What does this change imply about you? It implies the same potential as found in the rest of nature. Each day the sky demonstrates its power – clouds form and disperse, rain and snow descend and evaporate, windstorms whirl and depart. From where does the sky's power arise? It is already there within the sky. Your power is already there for your use. There are three secrets to increasing it.

The first secret is that you lay claim to your energy potential by trusting it. It resides inside and beside you. You have your intrinsic resources in conjunction with those that nature provides. Further

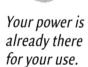

Your power is already there for your use.

elaboration is hardly necessary. You live amidst energy fields, the food and liquid you ingest are energy, the thoughts you think are forms of energy that instigate actions which in turn uses your body energy. Whether or not you call upon and make claim to these energy sources is your privilege. The qualitative difference in your life that gives you the edge over the ways other people use their energy is the experiential knowledge acquired by testing your energy resources. You have learned where and how to deploy it.

The second secret is that your energy always has the innate power to become more vigorous. No matter how small an energy change you feel, it demonstrates ability. You passed from a condition of indifferent energy to a phase of organized vitality. People get confused on this point. To often they measure their slight change against some imagined, abstract, gigantic accomplishment and get discouraged by the discrepancy. Organic growth is incremental so that you can integrate the change. No matter how small or great the change, you have proved the possibility. Your change shows an increase in your power, you are stronger than before. On the other hand, a change in energy – particularly an attitude change – can provoke enormous increase in your life force in a very brief period. The key is the recurring verification of dynamism.

Where and how change comes about is directly related to the intelligent use of your life force. When this power is activated it gets stronger. There is nothing capricious about your endeavor. You start with the intent of upgrading your vital force, then concentrate on one or more of your six resources of attitude, diet, breath, movement, rest, and solitude. Your body and mind are then shaped into those energy patterns that match your aim.

The third secret is that organized, organic change yields awareness of its power and its results. Awareness beckons control. Expanding your awareness produces versatility of control. Gradually you become aware of your power through its activation. Using your energy skillfully you develop familiarity with the art of wellness. You are unhappy when you think you have little or no power to change your body or mind, or if you feel your power but cannot control it. If you deny that you have any power over your life, just ask yourself what emotion recurs in your life most often. The presence of emotion belies your denial of power. Emotion, positive or negative, is power. Even recurring thoughts like, "I can't change," "What's the use?" "I always fail," "I'm no good" demonstrate power because they produce the intended result. In other words, whether you deny that you have power or whether you affirm an abundance, you fulfill your prediction.

The results of your judgment about your power always proves out. Why? Because the admission shapes the energy of your future. Your energy changes in accordance to what you intend. Your judgment about your potential actualizes your power in that direction. When you voluntarily quit an initiative change, you allow the thought of quitting to override the thought of persisting. Otherwise does quitting occur? The fits and starts that seem to characterize so much of your efforts are necessary experiences for you. They help you find out where your temporary limits are, what your interests are, and how you want to shape your future. The time finally comes when you stop limiting your energy, when you put your constrictions to rest. Then no self-imposed boundary will dampen your learning. Those fits and starts will unite and the quality of your life will never be the same.

PRACTICE SESSION

The Sixty-One Points Exercise

The ancient Himalayan yoga exercise of Sixty-One Points is very special. It refines your body awareness and opens the energy of your body-mind complex to your control. It will also develop your creative power; biofeedback research showed that this exercise increased theta activity. Over the months of daily practice, your intuitive awareness will develop so that you can detect body imbalances and correct them.

- LIE DOWN exactly as you do for progressive relaxation. It would be to your advantage to place a small pillow under your head for comfort and a dark cloth over your eyes to eliminate distractions from light.

- CLOSE YOUR EYES and breathe diaphragmatically for a few minutes until you feel quiet and relaxed. You are going to consciously travel throughout your body in a systematic manner, pausing at 61 key spots for two seconds each.

- **FIRST, FOCUS YOUR ATTENTION** at the spot between your eyebrows:#1. Stay there and at each point for two seconds.

- **NOW MOVE YOUR ATTENTION** to your throat pit:#2.

- **NEXT MOVE YOUR ATTENTION** to your right shoulder: #3.

- **NOW MOVE YOUR ATTENTION** to your right elbow joint: #4.

- **MOVE YOUR ATTENTION** down to your right wrist joint on the outside: #5.

- **MOVE YOUR ATTENTION** to the tips of your right thumb, # 6, your index finger, #7, your middle finger, #8, your ring finger, #9, and your small finger, #10.

- **NEXT MOVE YOUR ATTENTION** to the inside of your right wrist: #11.

- **NOW MOVE YOUR ATTENTION** to the inside of your right elbow joint: #12.

- **MOVE YOUR ATTENTION** up to the right shoulder joint: #13.

- **NEXT MOVE YOUR ATTENTION** to the throat pit again: #14.

- **NOW MOVE YOUR ATTENTION** to the left shoulder, #15 and move down the outside of the arm to the elbow joint, #16, the wrist, #17, the tips of the thumb, #18, index finger, #19, middle finger, #20, ring finger, #21, little finger, #22.

- **NOW MOVE UP** to the wrist joint on the inside: #23.

- **MOVE YOUR ATTENTION** to the elbow joint on the inside: #24.

- **MOVE YOUR ATTENTION** to the left shoulder:#25.

- **NOW MOVE YOUR ATTENTION** again to the throat:#26.

- **MOVE YOUR ATTENTION** to the center of the chest, #27, to the right breast, #28, back to the center of the chest, #29, to the left breast, #30, back to the center of the chest, #31.

- **MOVE YOUR ATTENTION** down to the navel: #32, then three inches below the navel:#33.

- MOVE YOUR ATTENTION to the inside of the right hip, #34, the inside of the right knee joint, #35, the right ankle joint, #36, the tips of the large toe, #37, the second toe, #38, the middle toe, #39, the fourth toe, #40, and the little toe, #41. Return up the leg on the outside to the ankle, #42, the knee joint, #43, the hip joint, #44, to the spot three inches below the navel, #45.

- NOW MOVE through the left leg in the same manner, # 46 through #57, the spot three inches below the navel.

- NOW MOVE YOUR ATTENTION to the navel, #58, the center of the chest, #59, the throat pit, #60, and the space between the eyebrows, #61.

Then exhale from the crown through the body and out the feet, returning inhalation up from the feet through the body and out the crown for ten breaths.

Your objective is to refine the body travel to that stage where it is smoothly accomplished without any distractions. As you get familiar with the 61 points, coordinate it with breathing. If you get sleepy, stop the exercise. Do it only when you are fresh and attentive. If you are combining this exercise with others in this book, do the 61 points after your breathing exercises and before your meditation.

NOTE: This exercise is available on The Wellness Tree cassette tapes. See order page.

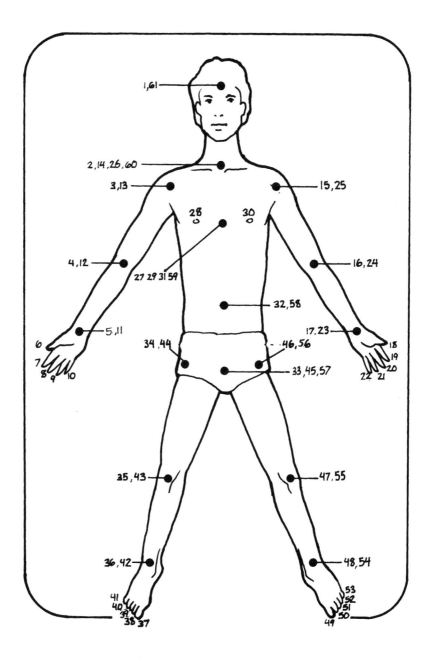

PART 4

BRANCHING OUT AND FLOWERING

CHAPTER 10

The Future of Wellness

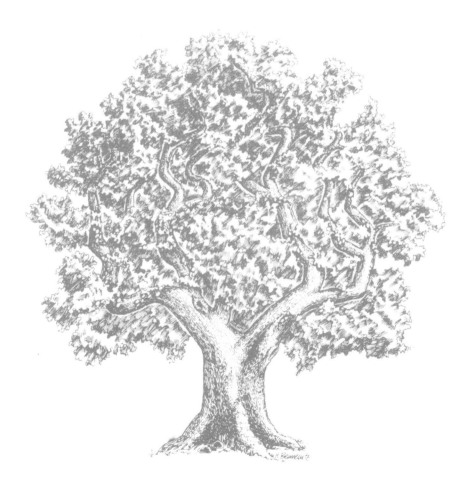

S CIENTISTS ARE ON THE BRINK of hypothesizing, or at least suspecting, that energy and consciousness interface. Twenty-five years ago, the contributions of biofeedback research startled us into realizing that we could consciously control our seemingly non-controllable bodily systems like heart beat and blood flow. Prior to that, medical textbooks assured us that the entire autonomic nervous system worked only on automatic pilot, that our central nervous system, our endocrine system and our immune system were virtually autonomous, and that the vast majority of internal functions were not on speaking terms with human will or imagination.

Today, while the scientific recognition for cross communication has unevenly achieved "official" status, we can, nevertheless, utilize these thresholds. The evidence is mounting that all our assumed autonomous systems readily communicate with each other. The brain and the systems of the body have molecular conversations about anything and everything that is occurring in their territories. While the terrain of body, brain, and mind differ, their borders are not the resistive guards they were previously assumed to be. The practical possibilities of body-mind communication are gradually dawning for professionals and laymen alike. Becoming aware of our ability to influence internal changes in our energy systems is valuable, if for no other reason than to banish the long-running superstition that separates mind from body. If it were not for articulate pioneers like Neal Miller, Elmer and Alyce Green, Barbara Brown, Candace Pert, Ernest Rossi, and others, we still might not appreciate that what really counts in human behavior and in wellness is what is inside.

The technology of biofeedback corroborates the individual's natural capacity for self-healing and independence and attests to the fact that consciousness is the fulcrum of well being. In considering your person from an energy perspective, biofeedback, meditation, and visualization confirm an exciting area to explore: the unrestricted, self-directed possibilities of intervening in the internal dynamics of your life force. The energy intent of your thinking and feeling makes all the difference to your body. As we have seen, how you assess yourself is much more than an idea in your head; it is a force that modifies your body's self-regulatory processes. There are far too many healing stories – clinical as well as anecdotal – that vouch for self-directed capacities unacknowledged in traditional medical texts. While one would be hard pressed to find a single chapter on healing in those texts, it is obvious that healing does occur, sometimes in very strange ways, as we will see in the following pages.

MIND YOUR MATTER: PLACEBO THINKING

A few years ago the British Government eagerly introduced its controversial list of drugs available by prescription from the National Health Service for the public. The Ministers of Government insisted that these products would suit the needs of all patients having the listed illnesses, nothing else would be necessary, and no patient would suffer unduly. The underlying premise supporting this statement was the claim that the healing of patients is solely a matter of pharmacology. The magic is in the pills; the disposition of the recipient is of no consequence.

Not long after this proclamation, a North London physician recalled the visit of a pharmaceutical representative. The salesman extolled the healing properties of a new drug to treat gastric ulcers.

He showed charts that indicated 75% of patients in a certain trial had their ulcers healed by this drug while in another trial only 41% were healed by a placebo – a sugar pill. While the rep continued to point out the obvious superiority of his product, the physician kept pondering the 41% who had their ulcers healed by a completely inactive preparation!

The placebo effect is viewed as a nuisance by the medical profession. Researchers and physicians can ignore its influence, but that dismissal will not banish its lurking, unpredictable presence. It occurs when you least suspect it, and in every branch of medical practice, conventional or otherwise. How can one understand its workings? How does one categorize it? If one wants to be meticulous and follow out scientific procedures, then what guidelines are available for this seemingly untidy parcel of influence? Is there any way one can rely upon them with clinical consistency? The answer is no, because a placebo is based not upon a quantifiable substance but upon human intent, what can best be called a form of creative self-management.

THE VERSATILITY OF PLACEBOS

Like the proverbial Murphy, placebos play havoc with the best-laid plans. They especially pay little heed to statistics.

A woman with severe nausea and vomiting was given all the standard remedies to no avail. She was finally told by her physician about a new "wonder drug" which guaranteed a cure. Exhausted from her ordeal, the woman eagerly took the drug with great hope. Twenty minutes later her nausea vanished, the vomiting ceased, and all her gastric tests results read normal.

The substance given to the sick woman was syrup of ipecac – a drug used to induce vomiting.[2]

It would seem that the woman's own self-regulatory dynamism, her belief system, and her wish to get well completely overrode the specific chemical impact of ipecac and produced the opposite effect.

During World War II, Henry Beecher observed that among all the soldiers wounded on a Pacific beachhead, only a quarter of the seriously wounded required medication for pain. The same tissue damage and injuries would require much stronger medication if civilians suffered them back home. Beecher postulated that the meaning of the pain changed due to the ensuing circumstances. For the soldiers, the serious wounds were a ticket home, out of the war. For the civilian, a serious accident meant social burdens like hospital bills, loss of job days, recuperation away from home, and more. Interestingly, Beecher also found that soldiers with less serious wounds felt more pain and required more medication because they knew that they would be returned to battle.[3]

There is also no reason to suppose that placebos are always good guys:

Harry was an investment banker. He dealt with statistics in all the financial planning for his clients. He believed in statistics; he loved percentages. One day Harry's physician informed him that he had prostate cancer. Harry carefully studied the medical statistics for his disease and learned that the percentages indicated no possibility of recovery. He told his physician that unless he died, his career would not make sense. Harry remained logical and faithful to the statistics. He had a small funeral.

Is this placebo thinking in reverse? Did Harry's determination to be statistically correct have a negative influence upon his eventual outcome? Don't we do that too? Take the common cold, for example. We all speak of "catching" colds. We speak of "the season" for them. They "run" through families until everyone "gets" them. Then there is the attack by the "office flu bug" lurking about on a chilly day. Ordinarily we are told to treat them with nasal decongestants, antihistamines, cough syrup, even, strange as it may seem, vitamins. Is the presence of tiny, infectious agents the cause for being afflicted with a cold of the flu? Why do some people "catch" them and others not? Could there be a meaning to my cold that is more than the proximity of infectious agents? Could my lifestyle make me susceptible to a host of noxious microorganisms that otherwise would not bother me?

SURGERY AS PLACEBO

In the 1950s, ten thousand people were involved in a new surgical procedure to relieve chest pain caused by coronary heart disease. The procedure required opening the chest and tying off an artery. Most of the patients (65–75%) reported vast improvement: pain was lessened and they had an increased tolerance for exercise. Some physicians remained skeptical about this "internal mammary ligation" however, so a blind study was undertaken to test its effectiveness. Candidates for the operation were randomly assigned into two groups. The first group received the new operation. The second group had a sham operation: incisions were made in their chests and they were then closed up without any other procedure being done. Post operative care for both groups was identical. No one except the surgeons knew which group had the real operation.

The therapeutic results were virtually the same for both groups, except the placebo group showed better improvement after six months.[4]

THE BEWILDERING CAPER OF MR. WRIGHT

The gentleman lay in the hospital bed on borrowed time. Riddled with lymphosarcoma, his neck, armpits, chest, and abdomen were distended with baseball-sized tumors, and he could breathe only with mechanical assistance. His spleen and liver were grossly enlarged, his chest daily drained two quarts of foul-smelling liquid. All medical treatments were deemed ineffective and the merciful prognostication was that he had two weeks to live. When this tragic picture of malignancy learned about a study, he gasped pleadingly to be included in a new trial with an experimental drug called Krebiozen. But the clinic wanted patients with at least three months longevity and Mr. Wright's febrile condition made him ineligible.

Quite against the rules of the Krebiozen committee, Mr. Wright was included with the twelve other subjects in the study as a gesture of kindness. He was given an injection on Friday. Expecting him to be dead on Monday, his personal physician was astonished to see Mr. Wright walking around, cheerfully chatting about his good fortune to whoever would listen. His tumors had regressed to half their size, even though they had been totally unaffected by earlier radiation treatments. Now it was decided that he would have three Krebiozen injections weekly. Ten days later, with the dumbfounded staff looking on, "terminal" Mr. Wright sauntered out the hospital doors and flew off in his plane.

As the weeks passed, other testing clinics reported no positive results with Krebiozen. Mr. Wright, who enjoyed unsurpassed good health for two months, read the newspaper reports and became very disturbed. He shortly reentered the hospital with a full relapse. His body resumed his original pathology exactly; all the horrible symptoms returned.

His physician, feeling he had nothing to lose, took creative advantage of the situation. He informed the despairing patient that his relapse was due to the fact that the Krebiozen in the original injections had deteriorated due to faulty bottles, but a new, super-refined, double-strength batch would soon arrive for him. Delaying a few days to gain effect, the physician finally injected the ecstatically optimistic man with the doubly potent, 'wonder drug' – plain water!

This time Mr. Wright's recovery eclipsed his first one. The secret water injections continued for a few days and Mr. Wright departed the hospital, a picture of health as he waved farewell from his plane.

Symptom-free for over two months, Mr. Wright read one day in the local newspaper that the American Medical Association declared Krebiozen to be a worthless drug in the treatment of cancer.

A few days later Mr. Wright was readmitted to the hospital. In less than 48 hours he was dead.[5]

What was the placebo in the saga of Mr. Wright? Was it in the bottle or in his head?

PLACEBO HEXES

Physicians claim that disease is caused by malfunctioning cellular processes, a breakdown of the body machine. The medical model claims that disarranged molecules produce aberrant illness. Proper procedure means gathering data about the functioning of the body through tests in order to pinpoint the deranged molecules for treatment. Exceptions to this model – afflictions not in standard textbooks, for example – indicate that the data is insufficient, but not the model. It is believed that eventually all ailments will yield to molecular analysis, and an appropriate molecular intervention, such as a new drug, will restore health.

For two weeks the newly graduated physicians, half way into their year of internship, had submitted and resubmitted the new patient to every conceivable test, from x-rays to blood analysis. In six months, the patient had lost 50 pounds; he was emaciated and weak. His admission designation was cancer, but not the slightest hint of pathology could be found on any examination. Here was a 'normal' elderly man without any real disease, yet he was truly dying before their eyes. The man, a simple farmer, was proving an exception to every rule; all medical analysis indicated that his systems and organs were functioning normally. Exasperated, one of the physicians finally told the man that he was dying and confessed that neither he nor his colleagues knew why. The farmer consoled the physician, absolving him of concern. "It's not your fault," he told them, "I've been hexed."

The unscientific explanation further unfolded. Some months before admitting himself to the hospital, a personal enemy of the farmer hired a local shaman to put a curse on him. The shaman obtained a lock of the farmer's hair from the floor of the barbershop and used it to put a hex on the farmer. Later, the shaman told the farmer and his adversary that the spell was cast and the farmer would now die.

The amazed physicians listened to the story and went away to strategize. They came up with a plan. One midnight during the quiet weekend, with hardly a soul around, they wheeled the farmer surreptitiously down the corridor into the examining room and locked the doors securely. The room was in darkness except for the eerie blue light radiating from the center of the table. One of the physicians produced a pair of stainless surgical scissors and slowly moved toward the transfixed, patient. Solemnly he cut a small lock of gray hair, dropped it into the flame, and announced that as the fire burned the hair, the hex upon the man's body would be destroyed. They all watched as the hair sizzled and turned to ash in the soft blue flame. The farmer was cautioned that should he reveal this ceremony to anyone, the hex would avenge itself upon him again, even more strongly than before. He was wheeled back to his bed and the antibiotic methenamine tablet was extinguished.

The following morning the "terminal" patient ordered a triple breakfast. Every meal thereafter was a double helping of food. Some days later the ebullient, fattened farmer departed from the hospital never to return.[6]

Did spontaneous disease meet spontaneous science and produce spontaneous remission? Was this another bizarre episode in Murphy's law of placebo thinking? Perhaps the physicians were confirming the admonition of Dr. Armand Trosseau that "you should treat as many patients as possible with new drugs while they still have the power to heal?"

THE MARX BROTHERS PLACEBO

Norman Cousins, the former editor of *The Saturday Review*, and Adjunct Professor at UCLA's School of Medicine had some interesting bouts with illnesses and developed some interesting cures.

At the age of ten Cousins was misdiagnosed and sent to a tuberculosis sanitarium for six months. Left on his own for the most part, he and some other patients formed into a group. They all assumed that they would soon return to their normal lives and planned accordingly. The confident, optimistic group stood in contradistinction to the other patients who resigned themselves to their prolonged and fatal destiny. Cousins' group even sought out recruits upon their arrival before the "bleak brigade went to work," convincing new patients that they would not recover. The boys in Cousin's group demonstrated "a far higher percentage of 'discharged as cured' outcomes than the kids in the other group."

At age 39, Cousins developed an arthritic and rheumatoid-like disease of his connective tissues, diagnosed as ankylosing spondylitis. He treated himself with strong doses of positive emotions and hours and hours of humor – Marx Brothers movies and reruns of Allen Funt's Candid Camera. He was soon well again.

Later, in his sixties, Cousins had massive heart failure. Again, he self-administered the wisdom of his humor medicine. He was back on the tennis court within a couple of months.[7]

Four heart specialists associated with Cousins noted five factors in his self-therapeutic attitude:

1. The absence of panic in the face of grave symptoms.

2. An unshakable confidence in his body's self-healing ability.

3. Irrepressible cheerfulness.

4. A "partner relationship" with his physicians.

5. A firm focus on creative and meaningful goals, which made his recovery and life worth fighting for.

In both instances of his rapid cures, many physicians informed

Cousins that he had been misdiagnosed. In their minds, positive attitudes and emotions could not affect the biochemistry of the body to facilitate rejuvenation. Cousins was cured, but he still remains suspect. For their part, physicians would be puzzled with his remark that the "placebo is the doctor who resides within."[8]

Most physicians are taught to think in terms of numbers, and so, like Harry the investment banker, they cannot find the answer to illness outside the corridors of statistics. They are often uncomfortable with unique, singular experiences of healing; more often than not, anecdotal evidence is disregarded. This is all understandable in light of the fact that the profession teaches its apprentices that the principal object of their study is not so much a living, organic, self-conscious being but more a mechanical, robotized, aggregate of molecules. "Physicians regard themselves as scientists and most of them believe that nothing is more unscientific than the notion that willpower or attitudes have anything to do with overcoming serious disease."[9] Recently a group of scientists met to determine whether or not monosodium glutamate is dangerous to health. After two days of testimony from consumers who described various adverse reactions to the additive from headaches to near-death experiences, spokesman for the scientists, Dr. Richard Wurtman of the Massachusetts Institute of Technology said, "There is no evidence orally consumed glutamate has any effect on the brain. The anecdotal experiences of individuals is superstition, not science."[10]

In their heralding of statistics, physicians and scientists often construct their own "Berlin wall," dividing themselves from the discoverable truths about life that will not necessarily lend themselves to the allopathic version of quantifiable science. Their commitment to the medical model, the molecular paradigm, forfeits their power of curious awareness and imagination that could release them from their limited viewpoint and reveal the awesome capacity of the mind to pursue and organize multiple modes of scientific truth.

In spite of the traditional disdain for placebos and anecdotal evidence, the significant import of the placebo is that it stands as irrefutable testimony that people have within themselves a certain self-healing dynamism, which can be mobilized and/or enhanced with appropriate conscious cues. Belief *can* become biology, intent *can* be converted into physiological reality, even if we do not yet comprehend the subtle strategies involved. Some things just work in spite of the left brain's ignorance.

These intriguing possibilities, however, are not a crusade to abandon chemical interventions. In this vastly changing world, we need to appreciate more and more that the human person is a multi-leveled energy being whose resources are accessible from different angles for growth and healing, not all of which can be reduced to the important molecular realm. The challenge is to pursue further the wonder of consciousness in human form. To this extent a more reasonable evaluation of the placebo could be appreciated along the lines of Norman Cousins' recommendation: the placebo is not so much a pill as a process, beginning with the patient's confidence in the doctor and extending through the full functioning of his own immunological system. The process works not because of any magic in the tablets but because the human body is its own best apothecary and because the most successful prescriptions are those that are filled by the body itself.

A NEW LOOK AT ENERGY

Akin to the philosophy of primary self-care espoused in this book is a medical viewpoint that is receiving controversial attention. This is a model for understanding the subtle, energetic structures of human nature that encompass an ecological sensitivity. Two recent, remarkable books – *Energy Medicine*, by Lawrence E. Badgley, M.D., and *Vibrational Medicine*, by Richard Gerber, M.D. – espouse this view. They explain their therapeutic approaches from an appreciation of the human multi-dimensional anatomy as complex and interrelated energy patterns. Each author brings, in his own distinctive way, a perspective that human well being is fostered by resonant energies.

Among current physicians, there are some that appreciate an understanding of the human person as a field of living energy and the generation of health and well being from multiple traditions. Dr. Dennis Chernin, for example, brings together in his practice a unique combination of nutrition, conventional medicine, and meditation. He has further broadened his medical perspective to include the remarkable tradition of homeopathy. This latter tradition has the enormous advantage over conventional medicine by understanding the permanent and unchanging in the phenomena of health and disease. Unlike conventional medicine, homeopathy assumes, like yoga science, that the human entity is fundamentally prone to self-healing and stability. Thus the homeopathic practitioner assists variously the innate, vital power of human nature to regain its stable balance in the individual.

When families head out for a vacation or holiday, homeopathy offers an almost comprehensive assortment of remedies for the typical accidents or momentary ailments that may be encountered. Dr. Chernin mentioned to me that the following would compose a handy first-aid kit: aconite, apis, arnica, calendula, carbo veg, colocynthis, ferrum phos, hypericum, ledum, nux vomica, and ruta. If you think your vacation area might meet with severe weather changes, sore muscles and bruises, cuts, indigestion, diarrhea, head aches, bone bruises, snake bites, travel sickness, and sprains, then a simple reading of homeopathic literature or the CD called *Homeopathic Resource* would educate the family to how to use these inexpensive, non-toxic remedies.

The promotion of optimal wellness and self-healing today is an uneven emergence of contributors whose collective vision accords with the growing awareness that we are indeed multi-dimensional beings of this living energy. When we keep in mind the Einsteinium contribution that views matter as an energy field, many of the energy-based therapeutic traditions can be better appreciated. Homeopathic remedies, flower essences, herbal ingredients, and gem elixirs, for example, charge the body with their specific vibration patterns to correct energy imbalances that show up as tangible diseases. Therapeutic touch, cranial osteopathy, and applied kinesiology, though distinct in their treatment forms, nevertheless presuppose the body as composed of interconnecting energy systems. Similarly, acupuncture posits energy channels, called meridians, throughout the body that guide the life force to perform its energetic functions at the physical level. In chiropractic treatments, the manipulation of the spinal column affects the spinal nerves so that their electromagnetic energy can function appropriately. Hydrochromatic therapy uses color tinctures in distilled water to charge the recipient with its chromatic vibrations for rebalancing one's energies.

In the area of investigative equipment, nothing arouses the heightened interest of hospital personnel more than the array of computerized body devises available today. The technological development of the CAT, CT, PET, and MRI scanners render possible, in particular ways, various cross-sectional, integral, and detailed views of molecular structure, cellular function, and tissue composition of the human body. The machines function, although quite expensively, as diagnostic imaging tools. It is particularly interesting that the non-invasive MRI device operates on the principle of resonance discernible in magnetic fields.

In step with this direction of biological resonance, there is another intriguing technology that has recently become available. This unusual invention, the Bio Energetic Transduction Aided Resonance – BETAR – scans the body for imbalanced patterns of energy, and, more importantly, delivers the proper resonance frequencies to balance the energy patterns currently restricting the healing process. It moves one giant step beyond the purely diagnostic capacities of conventional scanners. Whereas the MRI produces images of the structure and function of the body for diagnostic inspection, the BETAR combines its biological scanning system in biofeedback fashion with a monitored transmission of sound waves that relieve extraneous stress from the organic human complex. The BETAR reads the entire body's energy patterns and adjusts its frequencies within a range of 4Hz to 16Hz to restore and enhance the body's natural Shumann resonance. This resonance is the electro-magnetic pulsation of the earth, and also the pulsation of the human body in balanced health. The biologically active areas of the body responding to these frequencies are recorded by computer in conjunction with elapsed time so that diagnostic and recovery analysis can be appraised. The operator or health professional can observe the energy dispersal patterns occurring in the client. In a visual representation on a computer screen, the BETAR shows the discharge of the stored stresses that impede proper metabolic functions. The most frequent comment noted by clients after using the device is that they feel more relaxed and rested.[11]

Behind this usage of the word "energy" as applied to human vitality, my purpose has been to alert readers to the social tendency in modern health care practices to separate psyche and soma components of the one, unified, living human being. Over-emphasizing this division perpetrates an insurmountable dualism in the minds of health professionals and imbalances their approach to treatment. This dualism is passed on to clients and patients who then have a preconceived misunderstanding of the dynamics of healing and wellness.

The mind-body separation may be viewed as a problem in the communication of information. Put into the context of optimum wellness, we can ask some important questions. How does the semantics of thought affect cellular life? How does organic activity affect mental awareness? How do thoughts and body influence each other?

The various organs and processes of the body comprise an energy network of systems that are in constant communication among themselves. They supply, receive, and process information to and from each other. My heart, for example, does not pump independently of my rate of breathing, nor does my respiratory rate operate indifferently from my hormonal and emotional condition, which in turn is affected by the ideas and thoughts occupying my mind at the moment. Normal living is not one simple strategy for the mind and body but requires the constant intercommunication of many organic functions operating in response to each other. We live systemically.

The human being – a unified, self-reflecting, multi-leveled energy field of mind and body in relation to its environment – communicates back and forth between its parts by means of information transduction. (Transduction is a common phenomenon wherein energy is transformed from one code form to another without losing its value). Communication takes place within the individual's human energy field when energy transfers as conscious information. Typically the information-energy of thought converts into the energy of bodily matter and vice-versa. The body is always eavesdropping on its mind. Mental messages transduce via the brain to the body, shaping its cell life. The feelings and thought that you generate within your vast field of consciousness become the molecules that renew your body. You are constantly tailoring the body you want. It appears that the central integrator responsible for the cognitive and emotive functions of the mind interrelating with the biology of the body is the brain's limbic-hypothalamus system (LHS). This mutual arrangement does not imply, however, that the mind's energy is entirely confined to its body.

The purpose of technology in the context of wellness is not to replace human volition, but to function as an auxiliary to self-reliance. To this extent, reliance on many of our usual testing methods is misplaced. They measure parts of the body or mind in a static way, or disconnect parts of the human entity from other vital parts. The results given cannot then be accurate.

The treadmill test is a case in point. It purports to measure the amount of stress a patient's heart can withstand. Actually, it reveals what one's body can do in an artificial environment, while under pressure, in uncomfortable circumstances, and usually with an audience. Forgotten is the fact that the attitude in which the patient approaches the test has a bearing on its outcome. Some people are more apprehensive about a treadmill test than about a trip to the dentist. Prolonged fear, of course, inhibits cardiac efficiency. Mental stress, while it cannot be directly measured, directly affects the outcome of the heart's performance.

Equally important is the radical difference between a body that is being exercised and a body that exercises itself. The treadmill measures a body that is supposed to keep up with the machine. This is quite different from normal exercise. You might "flunk" the treadmill test, showing little endurance for sustained exercise, and yet have a heart that has the ability to sustain vigorous activity. The voluntary factor is crucial. Its denial on the treadmill makes the test misleading, at best. A better way to record the heart's capacity for exercise is by use of a Holter device. Since it records information while strapped around the chest, patients can use it while exercising on their own terms – doing their favorite exercise, at their own pace, in their usual setting, without pressure.

As long as we continue to think of ourselves as body and mind and emotions and spirit, we will continue to fail in testing, caring for, and healing the body-mind-emotion-spirit being that we are.

With all the modern improvements in health care, from vaccinations, microsurgery, organ transplants, and antibiotics to image scans, beta-blockers, artificial implants and radiation, one would expect a profound extension in longevity. Surprisingly, however, a forty-five-year-old male of today can expect, to outlive his counterpart of a century ago by fewer than two years![12]

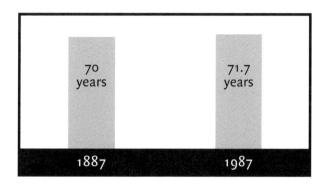

LIFESPAN OF A 45 YEAR OLD

We assume that the advance of medical technology promotes vigorous health and longevity, but wellness is not a matter of technology. As we have seen, it is the difference in the self-attitude that makes the difference.

....

"If we don't change our direction, we are likely to end up where we are headed."

– Old Chinese Proverb

....

OPT FOR HOPE

For some decades the researchers in mind over matter, as it is sometimes phrased, have known that we can exert personal control upon our internal states. We all have an innate capacity to intervene with our creative, subliminal minds in the regulation of all the physical processes of our body. From personal feedback experience, we can learn to manage the flow of electrical impulses in any nerve we choose. By the power of subtle volition and imagination, we can enlist appropriate dynamisms within the brain and its connecting organs to perform the objective stipulated by our intention. We can alter, for example, the blood temperature in the peripheral vessels of our hands and feet. This ordering procedure assumes precedence over the spontaneous or automatic physiologic activity that our bodies usually follow. The result is utterly compatible with the mind's intent. We are in control. An ordering sequence involving mind, brain and nervous system is at our beck and call, modifiable even further by experience and learning.

It is interesting that while most people learn to generate and recognize the correct mood or frame of mind for inducing these changes, they cannot say exactly how it occurs. The abstract proposition "I want my finger tips to warm" indicates the goal but is insufficient for obtaining the result. With intense concentration, you can rationally remind yourself of the goal and command your fingers, only to find that they get cooler. To actually obtain the desired changes, one must enter into a state of consciousness different from the patterns of thought and will. It is the subliminal dynamism of the creative unconsciousness that affects the internal ordering of the neurons and their communication to the extremities. Access into this subtle domain proceeds only with practice in tranquil awareness. It becomes increasingly clear that contemplation and meditation are indeed the next steps for humankind.

BEYOND THE LIMITS OF RATIONAL CONSCIOUSNESS

In the Spring of 1970 at the world's largest mental research center, the Menninger Foundation of Topeka, Kansas, an unusual series of experiments was conducted upon the range of human consciousness. It had been, and in some quarters of medical science still is, an accepted truism that human consciousness is quite restricted in its voluntary control over bodily organs and systems. The majority of physiological activities from the rate of cell repair to the movement of the digestive and heart organs is beyond the pale of rational control. The autonomic nervous system is not considered to be under the awake mind's direct and immediate utility. Most of the human body's activities and functions fall under the domain of the unconscious. Subjective purpose, in the sense of controlling both thought and body, is quite limited. There seems to be little credibility to anyone asserting that he could control his heart beat at will, accelerate or slow down the aging process, produce tumorous growths instantaneously or remain awake while permitting his brain and nervous system to sleep.

In order to discover whether these limitations were truly representative of consciousness' range of operations, the following experiments were conducted on one individual, Swami Rama, a yogi from the Himalayas, a physician himself and a holder of a graduate degree from Oxford University.

- THE LEADS OF TWO THERMISTORS (a sensitive detecting device that registers temperature changes at the surface of the skin) were connected to the subject's right palm. He predicted beforehand that he would alter the temperature between each side of his palm. Within a period of fifteen minutes, there was a simultaneous warming and cooling of the right hand, causing the "left side to become pink and the right side gray." The temperature between the sides was eventually 11 degrees Fahrenheit – an increase of 9 degrees over the original temperature. As the director of the experiment pointed out, "without moving or using muscle tension, the subject 'turned on' one of them (parts of the hand) and 'turned off' the other."

- WHILE REMAINING MOTIONLESS, and upon a given signal, the subject's heart beat slowed in less than 60 seconds from a pumping rate of 74 beats per minute to 52 beats per minute. At another time, the heart rate increased from 60 beats to 82 beats per minute in less than 8 seconds.

- IN AN EXPERIMENT to stop the heart and yet remain alive, the steady heart beat of 70 suddenly produced an atrial flutter wherein the heart rate average became 306 beats per minute for a 16.2 second interval. Actually, the length was closer to 30 seconds, because the technicians were surprised by the event of the dramatic heart alteration and conversed about it for some moments before fully recording the procedure. No blood can be pumped through the heart chambers when they open and close with such rapidity. The subject mentioned that he could sustain this performance for 30 minutes. This type of heart stoppage is often associated in cardiac arrest, producing unconsciousness, when "a section of the heart 'flutters' in oscillatory mode at its maximum rate, the chambers not filling properly, the valves not working properly and the blood pressure dropping."

🍃 SITTING MOTIONLESS, the subject "caused a 14-inch aluminum knitting needle mounted horizontally on a vertical shaft 5 feet away from him to rotate toward him through 10 degrees of arc." This exact direction and degree were requested by a member of the professional audience just as the experiment began. The experiment was immediately repeated with the same results.

🍃 ANNOUNCING THAT HE WOULD sleep for exactly 25 minutes, brain wave detecting equipment was connected to the subject's head, and thus monitored and verified the sleep state. Upon awakening at the precisely predetermined minute, he repeated the conversations of everyone in the room that took place during his sound sleep. He also accurately described the various activities that staff performed in other rooms while he was sleeping.[13]

In addition to these laboratory scheduled experiments, the same individual, in a less formal setting, performed the following:

🍃 HE RADIATED A FORM OF light energy, approximately 9 inches in diameter, from the center of his chest. A Polaroid photo was taken of the event "in which most of his chest was obscured by a disc of pale pink light."

🍃 IN A CASUAL CONVERSATION about tumors with the director of research at the Menninger Foundation, the subject asked the director to place his hand at a certain point on the subject's body. The director felt a lump under the skin resembling a moveable cyst. Then, on call, it simply vanished. He repeated the same congestion of cells at another part of his body which the director ascertained by touch. It also disappeared on call. On one occasion, a biopsy was obtained of two tumor-like formations, one on each forearm. The report of their analysis was exactly as the subject predicted: on one forearm the tumor was benign; on the other it was cancerous. They both receded on call.

🖋 BY THE SOFTEST TOUCH, the subject caused the middle portion of a solid piece of wood, a 12-inch ruler, to fracture into pieces. Similarly, using a metal-edged ruler held by the ends by two people, the subject merely pointed his index finger at the center part of the wood in a slow, downward motion, causing the wood to split apart and the metal edge to twist.

🖋 A CLINICAL PSYCHOLOGIST entered the subject's office for a visit. She was told to ask any four questions about any topic of her choice. After her initial surprise, she asked the subject four distinct and unrelated questions. As she finished asking the last question, the subject handed her a folded piece of paper upon which were written the four questions and his answers. He had written these sentences before she came to his office that day.

What is of special note here is the manner in which the majority of these experiments were accomplished. The intentional process whereby consciousness achieved the desired effects proceeded without the customary use of the laws of physics which govern mechanical activity. To alter, for example, the blood flow in the palm of my hand, certain causal relations are detectable empirically among the nerve fibers and members of my body to produce this result. Yet in most of the experiments mentioned, the effect took place at designated portions of the body that, in terms of its volitional occurrence, goes unexplained biologically speaking. Exactly how this force operates upon organic, human matter exceeds the conventional methods for empirical detection. In other words, Swami willed it and it happened. End of story. When asked by scientists how he was able to learn these abilities, Swami Rama said he owed it all to his practice of meditation.[14]

Swami willed it and it happened.

In this regard, Dr. Gordon Mayfield, a professional holistic practitioner, mentioned in a conversation to me that "... one of my primary goals is assisting people to take charge of their lives. It is essential to get in touch with one's inner self and have the ability to function in daily life from a balanced perspective in body, mind and spirit.

Through many years of study and work in the field of holistic health, I have found that the incredible power, stamina and focus that comes from the practice of yoga is literally life changing."

The purpose of Swami Rama's experiments was first, to force a revision of the cultural and scientific understanding of the boundaries of human consciousness, and second, to challenge a certain cultural despondency in our day. In the West, our century has produced the greatest abundance of material goods and the bloodiest wars of history. The technological prowess of our era surpasses the dreams of the industrial revolution, and yet there is more degenerative disease than ever before in medical history. Side by side with the advances of modern existence is a profound skepticism. The confusion and anxiety about the future leave people questioning the ultimate coherence of existence. A sense of the transience of life competes more strongly and easily today with traditional religious legacies that speak of eternal values. At the same time, the implication of these experiments reopens to culture questions about those telic clues within human nature that nourish and vindicate the progressive quest for the ultimate meaning of wellness.

LEVELS OF DEVELOPMENT

At this juncture, I propose a three-fold evolution that is discernible at least in recent decades, if not earlier. These three variable levels of body/mind development and regulation discoverable in recent Western human experience are not only repeatable in individuals, but disclose a certain open system feature about human nature.

Homeostasis. Built into each human is a certain biological stability that the body maintains under various internal and external conditions. Typically, the fixed patterns are temperature, pH level, heart rate, hormonal, immune, sleep cycle, blood pressure, etc. Whether the weather is blazingly hot or below freezing, the body attempts to hold its internal temperature, given slight variations, about 98.6°. Walter B. Cannon's famous publication *Wisdom of the Body* described this concept of homeostasis in which the human body has a memorized set of "right" values for its energy systems and the means to correct perceived imbalances. Medically speaking for most people, the energy patterns of level one are considered fixed and beyond the pale of modification or self-regulation. Thus, performance levels in life are expected and interpreted within this paradigm of homeostasis.

Homeodynamics. One can surprisingly reestablish the parameters of the internal systems and improve their performance levels. Physical exercise and aerobics enables its participants to lower their heart rate, tone up internal processes and external bodily dimensions, and cope with stressful circumstances more flexibility than previously assumed at level one. The 'right' values are modifiable. Thus, you can deliberately embark upon an improvement of your living energy for functional purposes. With training, your tonality, strength, and endurance improves your efficiency for functioning towards your personal goals.

Thanks to research and cultural participation in human development, our minds have became more receptive to the possibility of at least stretching us more ways than merely acceding to the 'fixed right' patterns of performance at level one. These training changes, however, are still accepted within a mindset that views them as adaptable within variable limits. The paradigm of level two shows a welcome flexibility, although we still view the apex of health as the absence of disease. As for the phenomena of placebo results and meditative self-control, these remain outside conventional possibilities as insignificant anomalies.

Homeo-reprogramming. Over the last twenty-five years, there has been an uneven recognition that we can go beyond levels one and two. The first level introduced us to an inherited set of energy patterns that foster and maintain our existence. The second level showed that these level one "normal" and "right" values are highly relative, for with training our biological components and emotional responses are much more adaptable than previously respected.

To some extent, we already knew at levels one and two that the person was self-conscious, self-organizing, and self-renewing. But we are both astonished and unsure, though intrigued, with the possibility that we can elicit a conscious "hands on" approach to designing our bodily and mental capacities and responses in an unprecedented performance.

The last few chapters have already cited various evidence that indicate the fixed energy patterns of biological, emotional, and mental regulation, control, and organization processes (levels one and two) are subject to conscious procedures that modify and expand them, even drastically. Surprisingly, the assigned functional energy patterns inherited from birth are not exempt from profound conscious influence.

The third level of demonstrated possibility points up the fact that the body/mind complex of level one and level two is, in reality, a flexible interaction of open systems of organized energy. While these open systems, including our autonomic processes, produce specific patterns of functional energy, they can be, with adequate training, profoundly re-configured to suit the utility of the intending agent. DNA may have hidden potentials awaiting conscious provocation The older paradigms of level one and two crack open and their energy reconfigures to that of optimal wellness.

Understanding the three-leveled interaction of consciousness reveals that the homeostasis, homeodynamics, and homeo-reprogramming principles of operation are within the nature of the human spirit.[15] The unifying context that serves, connects, and broadens these levels is the power of consciousness. Meditative states, biofeedback knowledge, autonomic self-control, spontaneous remission, healing images, laying on of hands, therapeutic touch, stress reduction, reframing dysfunctional embedded memory patterns and more are demonstrations systematically available to those willing to put time and energy into consciousness training. The task of life is less avoiding illness than pursuing and utilizing the action principles that foster optimal wellness. With our vital, conscious power we can grow from homeostatic absence of disease and aerobic conditioning to superb quality of life. By engaging the six-wellness resources as action principles, we can monitor our chosen directions, generate our energy, and enhance our life force toward optimal performance at any age.

Space is really not the last frontier; it's only a metaphor for the reaches of the mind.

PRACTICE SESSION

Creativity Exercises

Playfulness has much to do with creativity. Observe a child caught up in imaginary play: all business, pure creativity, but without any stress. Putting your mind in a playful mood can get around the blocks we adults set up around new ideas. When asked to do something highly innovative, most of us insist we feel uncreative, but our blockage is due more to fear than lack of talent. Fear is a self-imposed prohibition that reigns by intimidation. When you are afraid, you stop yourself from examining a part of life that could otherwise nurture you. Ironically, fear has no substance; it is not a thing, a virus, an event, or a person. Fear is a viewpoint, a state of mind. Creativity is a power, a state of being. So let us use our state of being to upset that state of mind. Let's dissolve fear with play while we deal with the tricks and treasures in our mind.

Playtime #1: The mirage of fear.

Place a lined sheet of paper in front of you. Draw a line from top to bottom dividing the paper into two columns.

In the left column make a list of all the things you would like to do, try, change, experience, but that also stir fear in you. If, for example, you would like to start a conversation with an attractive person at the office but are a little afraid of the encounter, list it. If you have been thinking about taking a course but feel too embarrassed to enroll, list it.

Next, in the right column name the fear for each item in the left column. Request your mind to tell you specifically what kind of fear or blockage you feel for each item. Is it fear of rejection? Fear of making a mistake? Fear of success?

Finally, look at your list in a new way. Ask yourself some questions: How real is this fear for me? Am I justified in sustaining this fear? What ways can I come up with to dismantle it? Often we have fears that have run their course long ago. They are really dead, with only a semblance of form remaining, like corn stalks in late Autumn. By interrogating yourself about your fears, the balance of power shifts to you and the fear dissolves.

Playtime #2: Exposing the "Can't" Trap.

Take another sheet of lined paper and divide it down the center into two columns.

In the left column list all the things you would like to do but can't do for one reason or another.

In the right column, list why you can't do it. Is it because of lack of competence, time, money, and connections?

Now really scrutinize your reasons. Are you stopping yourself needlessly? Are there any circumstances on the list that you can alter? Look at the list often during the next few days and allow your subconscious mind to give you practical solutions to the problems.

Playtime #3: Simplifying life.

Take another paper and this time divide it into three columns. In the left column list all your activities during a normal week. List events for every hour of your day. It does not matter how important or trivial the activity, just write it down.

In the middle column list the amount of time spent on that activity. Be as accurate as possible.

In the last column list those activities that you could (1) eliminate, (2) trim down in time, or (3) give more time to. Be ruthless! It is a safe bet that if you can't find anything to eliminate, you are not being totally honest with yourself. You should be able to "find" some time for building your optimum wellness through exercise, solitude, breathing practice, etc.

Playtime # 4: Back to your future.

Sit quietly with your eyes closed and breathe calmly for three to five minutes. Imagine how you would like your life to be in five years. Project ahead in time, and in your imagination do the things you would like to be doing then. Bring all your senses to bear. Feel the feelings. See your surroundings. Smell the scents in that place. Notice the people who are with you. Note what you are wearing, what the weather is like. Feel the smile on your face. Allow an entire scenario to unfold before you.

Now write down a detailed description of this future life on a sheet of paper. But write as though you were penning a letter to a close friend; write as though everything has already happened, and with great detail. As you write, you are composing your future. Watch how it unfolds for you.

Playtime #5: Upside-down thinking.

Purchase a notebook. In it write all the unusual ideas that occur to you during the day. Put in it questions, new problems, fresh ways of looking at something, whatever strikes you as odd, curious quotes, projections, plans, interesting remarks.

Occasionally, read through your notebook. The juxtaposition of thoughts and images will produce upside-down thinking – turning your thinking on its head to get a new view. It prevents you from getting stuck in stale thoughts. Ask your mind what you can do to implement any of the ideas. Then sit back and wait.

CHAPTER 11

Relationship with Life

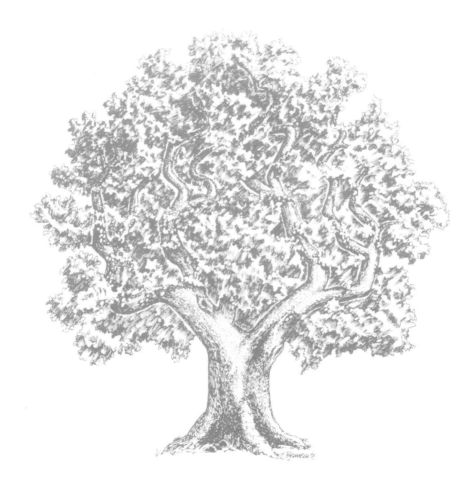

L IKE WAKING UP TO A NEW MORNING, our world is entering a new era. The information age is transforming people and continents. The geography of the cosmos, human potential, and its political ingenuity, reveal a vaster range of interpenetrating and interactive energy than we ever suspected. Global communication is part of our everyday awareness; nothing stays hidden for long. Private and public institutions are being forced to re-examine their purposes, becoming more fluid and experimental in their external structures. Organizations are revising their thrust toward consent and agreement, away from the old ways of command and obey. Countries are rewriting their constitutions because the old ways have outlived their value. People are demanding responsible ownership of their time and energy. From the arts to religion, to the sciences, former horizons are being pushed open to accommodate diversity and change.

All of these changes put a premium on learning. That is frightening for many people because learning implies that we will change our minds. But we can no longer rely exclusively upon our old maps of understanding, for, trustworthy as they are, they lack knowledge about the new discoveries on the horizon. In remaking the maps, we must relocate even the grid lines, for the old signposts are insufficient to guide us through the new fields of awareness. As we fill in and adjust the content of our new maps, we come upon old landmarks that have been covered over for quite some time. They are tragic places; we were never meant to venture there. The world has had enough suppression, now we must honor the unknown potential that nature and human ingenuity bequeath to us.

Today's people think thoughts and attempt changes in business and politics and lifestyle forbidden only yesterday. Who would have speculated that by 1988 eighty percent of the new businesses in America would be started by women? In 1989 who would have imagined the political turnovers of 1990 or 1992? And now we stand poised, as the world reconfirms itself for the third millennia.

CHOOSING YOUR WORLDVIEW

Like Copernicus in the Middle Ages, whose thought was not an extension of the current model of reality but a revolution in which he turned the world inside-out, we are on the brink of a new vision. These are times not for regret but for exhilarating, new work. We have our conventional paradigms and theories. Fine; now the challenge is to redefine and incorporate the new visions into the fresh paradigms and theories, temporary though they may be. New myths need to be composed, and the difficult task of their interpretation and corporation into daily life becomes paramount, lest we lose the benefits of our wonder by ignoring its meaning. Wonder is possible whenever change is honored and appreciated.

....

"Beliefs concerning the ultimate purpose and meaning of life and the accompanying worldview perspectives that mold beliefs of right and wrong are critically dependent, directly or by implication, on concepts regarding the conscious self and the mind-brain relation and the kinds of life goals and cosmic views which these allow."[1]

– Roger R. Sperry

....

Some people defend their worldview with a vigor that crowds out their sense of wonder. Others trap theirs through a fear of change. Their growth is mere repetition of the same structures and policies. When change is seen as an enemy, personal disaster is sure to follow. The wonder of new possibilities is frequently suppressed by those who need to defend the status quo. When the patient gets better after being told there is no hope for improvement, his physician may cast the improvement away as "spontaneous remission." When physicists are perplexed by cosmic discoveries that do not fit within the borders of their worldview, they may dismiss the new facts as statistically insignificant. The history of art, science, politics, and religion is replete with unorthodox views that were initially condemned.

A case or two in point: Newtonian physics, the paradigm of modern science, is a synthesis of principles and beliefs endorsed by scientists for more than two centuries. The scientific community was startled when its limitations became embarrassingly apparent after World War I. Novel experiments revealed phenomena at the microscopic and astro realms of nature that could not be accountable by Newton's theories. Scientific spokesmen assumed an unscientific, bureaucratic stance in their attempts to keep peers from communicating the new evidence. Journals refused to publish the maverick experiments because they were obviously defective articles exposing the failure of the proscribed worldview. Authoritative pronouncements by eminent leaders of the scientific community castigated them. In spite of all this, the new ideas won out. Forced by mounting evidence, a dazzling, pluralistic universe emerged from these continuing discoveries, giving birth to quantum physics and the theory of relativity. Nature had her ineluctable way: she was far more versatile in her wares than traditionally thought; energy diversified at more levels than suspected by the imagination of even the best Newtonian devotees.

Concurrently, in the field of electrical energy, another form of resistance unfolded. Thomas A. Edison, for all his inventiveness, confidently announced alternating current impossible to produce. Nature's electrical force could not be regulated in that manner, he declared. When Nicola Tesla, arguably the finest inventive mind in Western history, produced it simply and efficiently, Edison modified his statement to declare alternating current dangerous to life, and arranged to have it outlawed. Did his lucrative, direct current electrical company have anything to do with his proclamations? Tesla died in 1943, alone and discredited, bequeathing a treasure chest of inventions and theory books that are only belatedly appreciated and are now studiously combed for future applications.[2]

Near the Depression era of the 20th century, another adventurer managed to upset paradigms and policies on three fronts. With little formal education, Royal Rife invented the Universal Microscope utilizing prism lenses and over 5000 intricate parts. With his meticulously built instrument, he could magnify a specimen 61,000 times with unbelievable resolution, and enter sub-micro realms that were uncharted and unsuspected. To this day optical instruments are unable to come anywhere near this kind of enlargement; conventional electron microscopes kill any specimen observed. But Rife could inspect living bacteria and perceive their activities. Before his eyes, he could see that bacteria are pleomorphic, able to change into new forms according to their environment, thus challenging bacteriology textbooks which insist that bacteria are monomorphic, having only one form. Rife could illuminate micro-organisms and with properly tuned electromagnetic frequencies, destroy typhus, polio, herpes, cancer, leukemia, and other organisms in human blood with a painless three minute treatment. Alas, his inventions and research were vilified by the medical cartel, and Rife died a forgotten man.[3]

In the brief episodes described above, the eventual acceptance of the new discoveries did not banish previous knowledge. Rather, the new truths enlarged our understanding of nature and thus benefited humankind. Newtonian physics, for example, still functions quite effectively as a guide in our ordinary, three-dimensional world. And if, for argument's sake, you choose not to consciously involve yourself with your autonomic nervous system, nor accelerate your healing processes by augmenting your immune system, you can, most likely, still make it through the day. There are many truths, proven and suspected, that we do not hear about and whose absence will not interfere with our comfortable living. But there are marvelous discoveries that could advance and improve our knowledge of life and benefit health that are deliberately subverted because people do not like their worldview shaken, especially if the shaking threatens established prestige and income.

PARADIGMS ARE HARD TO GIVE UP

A good idea's successful career in society is never immune from vested interests. Everyone tries to capitalize on a popular theme even if it means counterfeiting its meaning or reverting to curious oxymorons. One manufacturer of chemical herbicides, for example, circulates an advertisement to farmers assuring them that their products "preserve our delicate environment." Another company produces a sticky-sweet confection that is a "natural health-food bar." It would be naive, as well as perilous, to absolve scientific decisions from cultural prejudice; ofttimes they are also weighted by economic and political power.

Rational convictions, beliefs, and assumptions, scientific or otherwise, are concepts relative to the experiences that generated them. The Newtonian worldview, for example, was essentially proposed upon a scientific basis. Its impact upon the culture and the historical era that accepted it, however, shaped its value into a cultural totality. A full blown myth arose for nearly three centuries: the cosmos is a vast machine inhabited by clever robots. While every thinking person has tacit ideas about the limits of the human mind and the frontiers of nature, a survey of the history of science and technology indisputably proves that the last word on either topic has not yet arrived. Like a perennial drama looking for a new cast of characters, truth moves on. At this writing, it appears that our delving into secrets of the universe verges near a startling future which endorses the dynamic interplay between consciousness and the cosmos.

....

"At the heart of science lies discovery which involves a change in worldview. Discovery, in science or the arts, is possible only in societies which accord their Citizens the freedom to pursue the truth where it may lead and which therefore have respect for different paths to the truth."

– John Polanyi, Canadian Nobel Laureate
Commencement address at McGill University, Montreal, June 1990

....

THE COMPASSIONATE MIND

Relating to life in its fullest means that we foster a humane attitude, one that views life as a journey to self-knowledge and self-expression. It also means we are not afraid to repair our mistakes. Life's challenge is the voluntary daily acceptance of ourselves while at the same time choosing a compassionate future for and with our bodies and minds. Compassion is a special quality of mind and heart in which we strive neither to dominate nor exploit, but to live, explore, and grow in rapport with the universe and all its inhabitants. It takes more fortitude to learn to live in accord with nature than to strike out at nature, especially when society assumes dominance to be a right. It is much easier to burn a rain forest for charcoal than to curtail the country's military budget.

The vision of compassionate living demands no less than a Herculean commitment to acknowledge the insurmountable grandeur of life in all its diverse forms, including its chaos and dissolution, and a willingness to endorse its new possibilities. A compassionate mind affirms difference, upholding diversity for its strength and its resources to insure the creation of a life-sustaining, new future. Compassion recognizes and memorializes loss but does not fear societal change any more than it fears the passing of the seasons. Compassion eschews the use or threat of violence as an instrument of policy in international relations. It decries the exploitation of the environment for short-term gains. A compassionate mind feels the need to constantly expand its responsibility for a global awareness – first for its own optimum wellness and then uniting in partnership with the world in which it lives for creating a new, humane future. There simply is no future unless we regard nature with the discerning respect accorded every living being.

> "To speak of the completeness and sufficiency of every man does not mean that men shall become more isolated and separated from one another. It means the possibility of a new kind of human community. If, for example, I do not need another in order to complete my own identity, I can see the other for what he really is in himself rather than simply for what he is that correlates with my own needs. I can now love and affirm him as a unique friend. Our social experience could then become multiplicative rather than just compensatory."[4]
>
> – H.R. Richardson

Dreams become realities when we aspire to the health and wellness they require. From where will the impulse arise to develop this kind of dynamic awareness? How does one generate the compassionate mind and access the energy resources for enabling its growth and maturity? Since thought precedes action, you might begin by pondering the following premises.

✎ YOU ARE UNIQUE, IRREPLACEABLE, AND SACRED.
Your spiritual essence is the same as mine but, ah, it shows up in so many delightfully different ways. Biochemical and anatomical variation are the rule. Your changing body is exclusive, yet you have a destiny that embraces more than your mind and body. Falter though you may, return to the quest that always vitalizes. Learn who you are from experiences and change who you want to be through your dreams.

✎ YOU ARE ULTIMATELY RESPONSIBLE FOR THE DESTINY OF YOUR LIFE FORCE.
If you do not claim your energies, then someone else – a preacher, a politician, a candlestick maker, will abscond with them. It is important for you to identify and defy organized cartels in religion, medicine, pharmaceuticals, art, and law that would imperil your human right to investigate richer visions of life.

✎ YOUR NATURE IS A DYNAMIC COMPOSITE OF BODY AND CONSCIOUSNESS.
This systemic network of bodily systems, emotions, memories, ratio-

nal and intuitive qualities, is, in principle, a unified whole. Any change in one area therefore affects the whole.

- ✒ OPTIMUM WELLNESS IS A FUNCTION OF EVERY ASPECT OF LIFE, NOT JUST THE PHYSICAL.
  The polymorphic diversity of nature is a metaphor for human energies yet to be manifest. Consciousness pervades your physical being to enable you to stay in touch with your body and emotions. Consciousness expands to be aware of your mental energy, your intuition, your environment, your neighbors. Communication fades if you do not take advantage of this arrangement.

- ✒ THE ENLIVENING FORCE FOR YOUR ENTIRE ORGANIC BEING IS CONSCIOUSNESS.
  Consciousness knows its matter. That means that your mind can be aware of your body at all times. Amnesia is only an interlude for you to dispel the fog of inattention to your self.

- ✒ YOU ARE MANY FORMS OF LIFE ENERGY: PHYSICAL, MENTAL, AND SPIRITUAL, AND THEY ARE ALL INTIMATELY RELATED.
  Your awareness is the vital element involved in whatever you feel, think, or do. View yourself as a whole being, otherwise your energies will decline into disarray and dis-ease.

- ✒ PERFECT HEALTH IS A MIRAGE, BUT THE PERFECTIBILITY OF WELLNESS IS YOUR BIRTHRIGHT.
  Growth and its cyclic rhythms always include breakdowns. I have yet to meet competence in any field that does not incur occasional lapses. Illness is undesirable, but it is not a matter for guilt. Instead, re-configure your stresses to advance to a new equilibrium of wellness.

- ✒ HEALING IS THE PREROGATIVE OF YOUR INNATE LIFE FORCE.
  Healing does not reside in any external agent, however adequately licensed. The notion that the center of the healing process is lodged with the healer is incorrect. It is lodged within each individual. The wise person knows how to summon and release its power. Healing, like happiness, is an inside job. In the midst of our country's tradition of freedoms, it is necessary today that freedom to seek the treatment of our choice be included in them.

🖋 AGENTS OF DISEASE ARE NOT ITS CAUSES.

Germs abound in and around you always, but the real issue is: What makes you susceptible to them? My grandmother cheerfully rushed to aid her neighbors whenever their children got sick or someone came down with a contagious ailment. She was never inoculated or immunized, yet she was also never seriously ill in her life. It is the disequilibrium of your energies that sets you up for illness; it is the way you treat yourself that determines the outcome.

🖋 YOUR BODY IS UNDER YOUR CONTROL.

Ordinarily, the range of the mind's awareness of its body is limited. With self-care training, you can gradually extend control and regulation of the entire bodily constitution and its autonomic processes.

🖋 SELF-MANAGEMENT IS EASY IF YOU START WITH THE SMALL THINGS FIRST.

Taking care of yourself requires discipline in little things. You get the sniffles, a slight infection, a cough that lingers, too much fatigue. It could be simple to manage, but if you ignore the clues or practice denial, you wind up paying the heavy price of serious illness later. On the mental and emotional plane, it is the same – start with the small things. If you find you are 'not in the mood' when a task needs doing, begin by doing something easy and tolerable, then quickly move on to something else. Your mind will alert you: brush your teeth, sweep the floor, pick up your papers, rearrange your desk. Get moving and keep ascending to more important things until you arrive where you wanted to be in the first place. Instead of fighting your mood, reshape its focus; energy yields to your direction.

🖋 YOUR BODY IS IN YOUR MIND.

The reason one can assume self-awareness and influence over the entire constitution is that the body is completely within the field of the mind's energy but the mind is not entirely within the body. Every cell knows what you are thinking.

🖋 YOU ARE COMPLETE, BUT UNFINISHED.

At the practical level of everyday existence, a human being is a complete, but unfinished, enterprise. The child becomes the adult. In adult growth and struggle, optimal wellness and maturity consists in discovering and actualizing the natural order of these imminent abilities. These functional powers are inter-dimensional, as it were, at the bodily, emotional, mental, and supramental levels. We neglect or abuse them at the peril of illness.

🍃 **YOU POSSESS ALL THE REQUIREMENTS FOR OPTIMAL WELLNESS.**
While our native biology and cultural education obviously conditions us, the applied knowledge of the fundamental principles of wellness allows the individual to improve, correct and even exceed society's expectations of humanity.

🍃 **LOVE WITHOUT BOLDNESS WON'T MAKE IT THROUGH LIFE.**
Love is, no doubt, the essence of life. But love cannot protect itself; it needs a champion. That is where your boldness comes in. Without it, your love wavers and you waste energy in pious dreams and "if only" lamentations. Boldness translates into a willingness to learn from experience and an attitude that diminishes fear to temporary caution. With boldness, love leads to wisdom.

🍃 **YOUR SPIRIT NEEDS MEANING IN YOUR LIFE.**
We live in an information age. Thanks to our computers, phones, and fax machines, we can communicate with anyone anywhere on this planet in a matter of seconds. We are bedazzled by the swift changes overtaking today's world and opening unprecedented opportunities in commerce, science, and art. Yet beneath the physical and emotional forms of stress in this technological age lies a restless agitation interfering with seeing what is real. "It is not the knowledge of things that is lacking in the contemporary spirit so much as the experience of things in themselves for what they are."[5] Our children grow up and away, promotions are fewer, the pension looms closer. We become anxious because we do not know what lies after our important, but transitory, work experiences. We must search for the real meaning behind all of life's events. Are we dampening or enhancing the fire of our life force – that fire which animates, illumines, protects, and inspires us to live a "little life with great, objective meaning"?[6]

🍃 **YOU ARE RESPONSIBLE FOR THE EARTH.**
If you are taking out more from the environment than you are putting in, your life is fraudulent. Put your life in order and the rest of the

world follows suit. Communicate with the chaos that surrounds you and restyle its energy. Make yourself accountable for your existence and inspire equitable demands of others. A global awareness of ecological wholeness must prevail so that our wounded planet will not continue to suffer for the exclusive profit of the few. In contrast with our indifferent desecration of nature for privatized commercial purposes, we need to reawaken our minds to honor our own affinity with nature. Without a deep connection to nature, personal spirituality is just another version of the "emperor's new clothes," a tight-fitting righteousness that ignores painful reality. In our collective attitude towards the earth, we act like immature children – always making energy demands upon our mother without the slightest notion of returning her favors. Any legitimate measure of human perfectibility must include a reverence for all life, human and otherwise, and the need to finally grow up.

HOW NATURE GETS SHORT CHANGED

One reason why Western religious rituals are impotent is their disconnection from natural experience. Christianity, Judaism, and Islam espouse no allegiance with nature. In fact, their theologies often perpetrate a utilitarian disregard for the earth, implying a suspicion about the noxious workings of nature's energies: what cannot be subjugated should be outlawed. This self-righteous mentality was seen in the aggressive condemnation of native nature ceremonials by the Christian missionaries and the governments that endorsed physical and cultural genocide.

Spiritual seekers, however, are mandated to enhance the cosmos, not from a biblical injunction, nor by a Supreme Court decision, but from a clear, unselfish commitment to the dignity of life. Human beings are nature's inhabitants. That is a self-evident truth that has been nearly abolished from public values. How many of us can see that the astonishing diversity of life in nature is a living metaphor for the creative splendor of consciousness? When we destroy the seas, the soil, the air, the plants, the animals, the forests, we shrivel emotional sensitivities and extinguish portions of our own self-growth. Removing these revelatory experiences of life diminishes our spirit;

banishing species forfeits opportunities for learning more about the very life forces that nurture us.

In our compulsion for progress we have abused earth's resources and plundered cultures. By a 'democratic' fallacy, we have considered earth's environment an arbitrary option. Our religious institutions have become morbidly introspective, dislocated from the sensual and sexual values of nature. Our industrial growth has caused our health to degenerate. By desecrating nature we have alienated ourselves from the creative processes that instill genuine wellness.

Both religion and commerce should be judged by their own severe standards: what have they done to nature for the success and expansion of their product? The magnitude of public greed and exploitation forces us to an irrevocable choice: we must live an ecological lifestyle. Only from an alignment with the biosystems of nature can we learn to integrate our human cultures with the vaster cosmos.

WORK FOR YOUR WELLNESS

The political changes of Eastern Europe in 1989 did not occur spontaneously. How many of our world leaders predicted them a year earlier? Everyone was caught unaware except those who worked painfully for the change. Citizens of the communist block said, "Enough of inhumane living."

Wellness models, like political schemes, are really strategies, practical guidelines for directing your otherwise random energy. It is unlikely that you will get very far without some purposeful structure, envisioned into a map, a manual, or a plan. Better models are proven by the principle of accountability: test the results. The best models leave room for a heuristic function, i.e., the recognition that intelligent probing of life may yield additional benefits. Make modifications on that basis. With such guidelines, you are less likely to fall prey to dogmatic insistence. A little pragmatism never hurts: if following the rules does not get me where I want to go why make them sacrosanct?

Like enticing cookbooks, models for wellness should offer various recipes to nourish your hunger. Taste them for awhile and note how you feel. People who claim no special rules still order their lives, or follow some regime, however inconspicuously. While the mind has a preference for order, it always hopes to find one that enlivens.

Optimal wellness is a heuristic model, adaptable to the relative energies of the person involved by the person involved. It postulates the theory that we are energy beings. It insists that our life energy can be enhanced, after almost any circumstances of abuse. It places human vitality into a primary context of self-responsibility that views the individual as a developing whole, a dynamic and harmonious equilibrium of energies and elements composing and surrounding it.

Optimal wellness proposes that amidst the inexorable flux of history and the ambiguities of an era, nature possesses an ordered set of dynamisms. When these are stimulated, self-awareness quickens. The more we learn to arouse and integrate our energies, the more our life force unfolds its further potential to consciousness for living well. The negative side is equally awesome: the less we engage our attention with our energies, the more we are subject to the whims of chance with our bodies and minds. In this regard, Andrew Weil remarks that "the primary responsibility for health is the patient's.... By way of encouragement, let me assure the reader that most of what I know about keeping myself in good health I did not learn in my training as a medical doctor. I learned it from observation of myself and others, from intuition and thought, and from my own experience."[7]

....

The world won't change until I change.

....

The Newtonian, mechanistic worldview brought us the machines of the Industrial Revolution. The inroads of quantum physics, with their technological inventions, show that we live in more than a one-story universe. The global transition of the 90's beckons us to render a meaning to our existence in its totality. The fragmentation and isolation of the past decades is vanishing, but we still have not recognized it as such. The greeting of Native Americans, *Mitakuye Oyasin*, is eminently true.[8]

The pluralistic universe of physics and politics invites us to pursue the marvels of bringing together the multiple levels of consciousness interfacing with the various energy configurations of nature and matter. We are about to create a new civilization. Consequently, among world citizens, there is a slow shifting towards a preference for experimentation and experiential validation. The formation of a lifestyle encompassing optimal wellness is a life-long process. Confidence emerges as self-initiating growth occurs. Trust in the life force produces an internal harmony that makes the world an enriching experience – a place of expanding vision that frees all beings to communicate their splendid differences for mutual enrichment.

AFTERWORD

I am honored
and extremely delighted
to end this work with the inspiration
of one whose life continues to model
the principles of vitality and love
prescribed within its pages.
My dear friend, Frederick Franck,
companion of Dr. Albert Schweitzer,
pictorial recorder of Vatican Council II,
originator and director of Pacem in Terris,
a garden of music, art, drama and peace,
writer of numerous luminous books,
artiste extraordinaire, whose works
enrich the world's museums,
authorizes with beauty
the last word.

MAY YOUR HEALTH BE STURDY, YOUR MIND CALM,
MAY YOU BE SPARED HOSPITALS AND COURTS OF
LAW, DOCTORS, SURGEONS, SHRINKS AND DENTISTS...
MAY YOUR LIVELIHOOD BE UNIMPAIRED. MAY
YOU BE SAFE FROM BEING BOMBED, MUGGED,
HELD HOSTAGE FOR WHATEVER MOTIVE, HIGH FLOWN
OR LOW SLUNG, AND PROTECTED FROM HARASSMENT,
BREAK-IN, TAPPING, ARREST, TORTURE AND DEATH
AT THE HANDS OF THOSE POISONED BY POWER,
AND UNSCATHED BY ALL THE OLD, PRIMITIVE
AS WELL AS THE NEW, SOPHISTICATED FORMS OF
BARBARITY... MAY WE ALL ESCAPE WARS
AND CONFLAGRATIONS, WHETHER CIVIL OR GLOBAL
AND BE UNESTRANGED FROM THOSE WE LOVE
MOST OF ALL: FROM OURSELVES...

May the Light that lighteneth Every One
come into this world pierce the darkness
of the age, so that
the tree of life may
survive and bring
forth new shoots!

frederick franck

NOTES

CHAPTER 2: ATTITUDE

1 C. Pert, *Molecules of Emotion*. New York: Scribner, 1997.
2 L. Player, *Medicine and Culture*. New York: Henry Holt, 1988, p. 9.
3 J. Goodfield, *Playing God*. New York: Random House, 1977.
4 Vernon Coleman, *The Health Scandal*. London: Sidgwick and Jackson, Ltd., 1988, p. 183.
5 R. Ornstein and D. Sobel, *The Healing Brain*. London: MacMillan, 1988, p. 182.

CHAPTER 3: BREATH

1 Phil Nuernberger, *Freedom From Stress*. Honesdale, PA: Himalayan Publishers, 1981, p. 4–5.
2 W.S. Bullough and E.B. Lawrence, "Accelerating and decelerating actions of adrenaline in epidemilotic activity." Vol. 210, 1966, p. 515–16.
3 Chandra Patel, *Fighting Heart Disease*. London: Dorling Kindersley, 1987.
4 Ester Sternberg, "Beyond Forklore: Stress Can Make You Sick," *Cerebrum: The Dana Forum on Brain Science*. Vol. 2, No. 1, Winter 2000, p. 136.
5 American Stress Institute, 1986.
6 Moshe Feldenkrais. *Awareness Through Movement*. NY: Harper & Row. 1977, p. 37.
7 For a fuller description of breath physiology see Justin O'Brien, *Running and Breathing*, Lakemont, GA: CSA Press, 1985.
8 The body has rhythms such as sleeping/waking, which are called the circadian cycles (from *circa-dies*, meaning about a day) and longer rhythms, such as the menstrual cycle, which are called

infradian cycles (from *infra-dies*, meaning longer than a day).

9 Alan Hymes and Phil Nuernberger. "Breathing Patterns Found in Heart Attack Patients," *Research Bulletin of the Himalayan Institute*, Vol. 2, No. 2, 1980.

10 Ernest Rossi. *The Psychobiology of Mind-Body Healing.* NY: Norton, 1986, Sec. II.

11 In Justin O'Brien's *Pioneer of Inner Space.* Fryeburg, ME: J. Appleseed &Co., 1989, p. 15.

CHAPTER 4: NUTRITION

1 Swami Rama, *A Practical Guide to Holistic Health.* Himalayan Publishers, Honesdale, PA, 1978.

2 M. Gerson, *A Cancer Therapy.* Del Mar, CA: Totality Books, 1977.

3 Barnard, N., "The Need for New Food Recommendations," *PCRM Update*, May–June 1991, p. 3.

4 Campbell, T.C., quoted in Attwood, C., "Summit in the Desert," unpublished.

5 Onish, D., *Dean Ornish's Program for Reversing Heart Disease*, NY: Random House, 1990.

6 U.S. Senate (Select Committee on Nutrition and Human Needs), *Nutrition and Health: An Evaluation of Nutritional Surveillance in the United States.* Washington, DC: Government Printing Office, 1975, p. 5.

7 In W. Dufty, *Sugar Blues.* New York: Warner Books, 1976.

8 F. Batmanghelidj, *Your Body's Many Cries for Water.* Falls Church, VA: Global Health Solutions, Inc., 1999.

CHAPTER 5: MOVEMENT

1 Dr. B. Stanford, *Sports Medicine*, Vol. 27, 1989.

2 "Biomedicine," in *Science News*, Vol. 137, p. 208.

3 P. Insel and W. Roth quoted in Justin O'Brien, *Running and Breathing, op. cit.*

4 J.A. Mortimer, P.J. Pirozzolo, and G.J. Natella, *The Aging Motor System.* New York: Praiger, 1982. p. 9. See also Thomas Honna, *Somatics.* New York: Addison-Wesley, 1988.

5 K. Pelletier, *Mind as Healer, Mind as Slayer.* New York: Delta, 1977.

6 Grateful acknowledgment is made to IRSA, The Association of Quality Clubs, for permission to reprint excerpts from *The Economic Benefits of Regular Exercise 1991*, and *The Benefits of Regular Exercise 1992*.

CHAPTER 6: REST

1 R. Edwards, *Coronary Case*. London: Faber, 1964.
2 Even in a peaceful country like Scotland more than fifty percent of the women over 65 require a tranquilizer to get to sleep each night.

CHAPTER 7: SOLITUDE

1 Andre Malraux, *Saturn, An Essay on Goya*. London: 1957, p. 25.
2 Evelyn Fox Keller, *A Feeling for the Organism*. Los Angeles: W.H. Freeman, 1983, p. 182.
3 *Ibid.*, p. 102.
4 *Ibid.*, p. 103.
5 *Ibid.*, p. 202.
6 See also Houston, Jean. *The Search for the Beloved: Journeys in Mythology and Sacred Psychology*. Los Angeles: Tarcher, 1987, p. 3–9.
7 *The Cloud of Unknowing and Other Works*. Trans. by C. Wolters. London: Penguin, 1978.
8 I. Bentov, *Stalking the Wild Pendulum*. VT: Destiny Books, 1988, p. 42–43.
9 See Justin O'Brien's "Meditation, An Inner Science" in *Christianity and Yoga: A Meeting of Mystic Paths*. London: Penguin, 1989, p. 60–69 and O'Brien's "The Development of Christian Meditation in Light of Yoga" in *Meditation in Christianity*. Honesdale, PA: Himalayan Press, 1983, p. 33–60.
10 M. Murphy, *The Future of the Body: Explorations Into the Further Evolution of Human Nature*. Los Angeles: J.P. Tarcher, 1992.

CHAPTER 8: CHOOSING LIFE

1 N. Cousins. *Head First: The Biology of Hope*. New York: Dutton, 1989, p. 253.

2 Elmer and Alice Green. *Beyond Biofeedback*. New York: Dellacorte, 1977, p. 210.

3 Personal communication with Tom Ferguson, M.D., editor of *Self-Care* magazine, 1991.

4 Marc Lappe. *When Antibiotics Fail: Restoring the Ecology of the Body*. Berkeley, CA: North Atlantic Books, 1986, p. 18.

5 R. Orstein and D. Sobel. *The Healing Brain*. London: MacMillan, 1988, p. 19.

6 Lappe, *op. cit.*, p. 17–18.

7 H.C. Neu. "The Crisis in Antibiotic Resistance," *Science*, Vol. 257, 1992, p. 1064–73.

8 *Journal of the American Medical Association*, Vol. 264, 1990, p. 1413–17.

9 Selye, Hans. *The Stress of Life*. New York: McGraw-Hill, 1956, p. 299.

10 *New England Journal of Medicine*, Vol. 325, 1991, p. 606–12.

11 *Ibid.*, Vol. 303, 1980, p. 1505–11.

12 E. Green. *Newsletter of the International Society for the Study of Subtle Energies and Energy Medicine*. Vol. 3, No. 1, Spring 1992.

13 Elmer and Alyce Green, *op. cit.*, p. 11, 116.

CHAPTER 9: RECREATING YOURSELF

1 Ellen J. Langer. *Mindfulness*. New York: Addison-Westley, 1989, Chapter 6.

2 E. Jacobson, *You Must Relax*. New York: McGraw-Hill, 1962.

3 P. Garfield, *Creative Dreaming*. New York: Ballantine, 1974, p. 44.

CHAPTER 10: FUTURE OF WELLNESS

1 Elmer and Alyce Green. *Beyond Biofeedback*. New York: Delacorte, 1977, p. 116.

2 R. Ornstein and D. Sobel. *The Healing Brain*. London: MacMillan, 1988, p. 79.

3 H.K. Beecher. "Relationship of Significance of Wound to Pain Experienced," *Journal of the American Medical Association*, Vol. 161, 1956, p. 1609–13.

4 *Ibid.*

5 B. Klopfer. "Psychological Variables in Human Cancer," in *Journal of Projective Techniques*, Vol. 21, 1957, p. 331–340.

6 Larry Dossey. *Space, Time & Medicine*. Boulder, CO: Shambala, 1982, p. 3–6.

7 Norman Cousins. *Anatomy of An Illness*. New York: Norton, 1979, p. 155–156.

8 *Ibid.* p. 69.

9 N. Cousins. *Head First: The Biology of Hope*. NY: E.P. Dutton, 1989, p. 3.

10 Associated Press, in *Star Tribune*, April 9, 1993, p. 2.

11 Peter J. Kelly. "The Betar and Its Scalar Detection System" paper presented, Second International Keely Symposium, 1989. *Omni*, Vol. 12, No. 3, p. 123.

12 See Ornstein, *op. cit.* for additional research.

13 Elmer and Alyce Green. *Beyond Biofeedback*. CA: Delacorte Press, 1977, p. 197–98, 200–201, 205. See also Elmer and Alyce Green, "The Ins and Outs of Mind-Body Energy," *Science Year: The World Book Science Annual*. Chicago: Field Enterprises Education Corp., 1974, and Elmer Green, "Biofeedback for Mind-Body Self-Regulation: Healing and Creativity." Kansas: The Menninger Foundation, 1971, p. 23.

14 *Beyond Biofeedback*, *Ibid.*, p. 209–11. See also D. Boyd, *Swami*, New York: Random House, 1976, p. 91–93.

15 I am indebted to Professor Otto Schmitt of the University of Minnesota for these insights.

CHAPTER 11: RELATIONSHIP WITH LIFE

1 R. Sperry. "Changing Priorities," paper presented at the Annual Review of Neuroscience, 1981, p. 1–15.

2 For a biography of this remarkable man see John O'Neill. *Prodigal Genius: The Life of Nikola Tesla*. Hollywood, CA: Angriff Press.

3 B. Lynes with J. Crane. *The Cancer Cure That Worked*. Ottawa, Canada: Marcus Books, 1987.

4 H.R. Richardson, *Three Myths of Transcendence*. Boston: Beacon Press, 1969, p. 111–112.

5 Laurens van der Post. *The Creative Pattern in Primitive Africa.* Eranos Lectures Series, No. 5, Toronto, CA: Spring Publications.

6 *Ibid.*

7 Andrew Weil, M.D. *Health and Healing.* Boston: Houghton Mifflin Co., 1983, p. 273.

8 "We are all related."

BIBLIOGRAPHY

ACHTERBERG, Jeanne. *Imagery in Healing: Shamanism and Modern Medicine.* Boston: New Science Library, 1985.

BADGLEY, Lawrence E. *Energy Medicine.* San Bruno, CA: Human Energy Press, 1985.

BATMANGHELIDJ, F. *Your Body's Many Cries for Water.* Falls Church, VA: Global Health Solutions, Inc., 1999.

BEARDEN, Thomas E. *Aids: Biological Warfare.* Greenville, TX: Tesla Book Co., 1988.

BECKER, Robert. *Cross Currents.* New York: St. Martin's Press, 1990.

BECKER, Robert and Selden, G. *The Body Electric: Electromagnetism and the Foundation of Life.* New York: William Morrow & Co., 1985.

BERRY, Thomas. *The Dream of the Earth.* San Francisco: Sierra Club Books, 1988.

BIRD, Christopher. *The Persecution and Trial of Gaston Naessens.* Tiburon, CA: H.J. Kramer, 1991.

BLACK, Dean. *Health At the Crossroads.* Springville, UT: Tapestry Press, 1988.

BROWN, Barbara B. *Stress and the Art of Biofeedback.* New York: Harper & Row, 1977.

BRYANT, Barry. *Cancer and Consciousness.* Boston: Sigo Press, 1990.

_____. *New Mind, New Body, Biofeedback: New Directions for the Mind.* New York: Harper & Row, 1974.

BULLOUGH, W.S. & Lawrence, E.B. "Accelerating & Decelerating Actions of Adrenaline in Epidemilotec Activity," *Nature,* Vol. 210: p. 715–6, 1966.

BURR, Harold S. *The Fields of Life.* New York: Ballantine, 1972.

CAPRA, Fritjof. *The Tao of Physics.* New York: Bantam, 1977.

CHOPRA, Deepak. *Unconditional Life: Mastering the Forces That Shape Personal Reality.* New York: Bantam, 1991.

_____. *Ageless Body, Timeless Mind.* New York: Harmony Books, 1993.

COLEMAN, Vernon. *The Health Scandal.* London: Sidgwick & Jackson, Ltd., 1988.

COOPER, Robert K. *The Performance Edge.* Boston: Houghton Mifflin, 1991.

COULTER, Harris L. *Divided Legacy: The Conflict Between Homeopathy and the American Medical Association.* Richmond, CA: North Atlantic, 1973.

COULTER, Harris L. and Fisher B. *Shot In the Dark.* New York: Avery, 1991.

COUSINS, Norman. *Anatomy of an Illness.* New York: Bantam, 1981.

_____. *The Healing Heart.* New York: Norton, 1983.

_____. *Head First: The Biology of Hope.* New York: Dutton, 1989.

DAEMION, Jonathan. *The Healing Power of Breath: An Introduction to Wholistic Breath Therapy.* New York: Avery Publishing Group, 1989.

DIENSTFREY, Harris. *Where the Mind Meets the Body.* New York: Harper Collins, 1991.

DONDEN, Yeshi. *Health Through Balance: An Introduction to Tibetan Medicine.* New York: Snow Lion Publications, 1986.

DOSSEY, Larry. *Beyond Illness: Discovering the Experience of Health.* Boston: Shambala, 1984.

_____. *Recovering the Soul: A Scientific and Spiritual Search.* New York: Bantam, 1989.

_____. *Healing Words.* San Francisco: Harper, 1993.

_____. *Prayer is Good Medicine.* San Francisco: Harper, 1996.

DUFTY, William. *Sugar Blues.* New York: Warner, 1975.

EDWARDS, Richard. *Coronary Case.* London: Faber, 1964.

FELDENKRAIS, Moshe. *Awareness Through Movement.* New York: Harper & Row, 1977.

GARFIELD, Peter. *Creative Dreaming.* New York: Ballentine, 1974.

GERBER, Richard. *Vibrational Medicine.* Sante Fe: Bear & Co., 1988.

GREEN, Elmer and Alice. *Beyond Biofeedback.* New York: Delacorte, 1977.

HANNA, Thomas. *Somantics: Reawakening the Mind's Control of Movement, Flexibility, and Health.* New York: Addison-Wesley, 1988.

HYMES, Alan and Nuernberger, Phil. "Breathing Patterns Found in Heart Attack Patients," *Research Bulletin of the Himalayan Institute*, Vol. 2, No. 2, 1980.

ILLICH, Ivan. *Medical Nemesis: The Expropriation of Health.* New York: Bantam, 1977.

JACOBSON, Edmond. *Progressive Relaxation.* Chicago: The University of Chicago Press, 1977.

_____. *You Must Relax.* New York: McGraw-Hill, 1968.

JANTSCH, Erich. *The Self Organizing Universe: Scientific and Human Implications of the Emerging Paradigm of Evolution.* New York: Pergamon Press, 1989.

JONAS, Hans. *The Phenomenon of Life.* New York: Dell, 1966.

LAPPE, Francis M. *Diet for a Small Planet.* New York: Ballantine, 1971.

LANGER, Ellen J. *Mindfulness.* Reading, MA: Addison-Wesley, 1990.

LaSHAN, Lawrence. *You Can Fight for Your Life.* New York: Evans, 1977.

LOWEN, Alexander. *Language of the Body.* New York: MacMillan, 1971.

LUCE, George G. *Biological Rhythms in Human and Animal Physiology.* New York: Dover, 1977.

LUTHE, Wolfgang (ed.) *Autogenic Therapy* (in six volumes). New York: Grune and Stratton, 1969.

LYNES, Berry with Crane, John. *The Cancer Cure that Worked.* Toronto: Marcus, 1987.

MACEY, Robert I. *Human Physiology.* New Jersey: Prentice-Hall, 1975.

MALROUX, Andre. *Saturn: An Essay on Goya.* London: Phaidon Press, 1957.

McCAMY, John C. and Presley, James. *Human Life Styling.* New York: Harper & Row, 1975.

McKEOWN, Thomas. *The Role of Medicine: Dream, Mirage or Nemesis?* Princeton, NJ: Princeton University Press, 1979.

MENNINGER, Karl. *The Vital Balance: The Life Process in Mental Health and Illness.* New York: Viking, 1963.

MESSEGUE, Maurice. *Of Mice and Plants.* New York: Bantam, 1974.

MOSS, Ralph H. *The Cancer Industry: The Classic Expose on the Cancer Establishment.* New York: Paragon House, 1989.

MOYERS, Bill. *Healing and the Mind.* New York: Doubleday, 1993.

MULLINS, Eustace. *Murder by Injection.* Staunton, VA: The National Council for Medical Research, 1992.

MURPHY, M. *The Future of the Body: Explorations in the Further Evolution of Human Nature*. Los Angeles: J.P. Tarcher, 1992.

NIXON, Peter G.F. "Stress and the Cardiovascular Systems," *The Practitioner*. Vol. 9, No. 226, 1982, p. 1589–98.

ORNISH, D., *Dean Ornish's Program for Reversing Heart Disease*. New York: Random House, 1990.

ORNSTEIN, Rorbert and Sobel, David. *The Healing Brain*. New York: MacMillan, 1988.

PATTEL, Chandra. *Fighting Heart Disease*. London: Dorling Kindersley, 1987.

PAYER, Lynn. *Medicine & Culture*. New York: Henry Holt, 1988.

PELLETIER, Kennith R. *Holistic Medicine*. New York: Delacorte, 1979.
_____. *Mind as Healer, Mind as Slayer*. New York: Delta, 1977.

PERT, Candace. *Molecules of Emotion*. New York: Scribner, 1997

PICARD, Max. *The World of Silence*. Washington, D.C.: Gateway Editions, 1988.

PRIGOGINE, I. and Stengers, I. *Order Out of Chaos: Man's New Dialogue With Nature*. New York: Bantam, 1984.

RUDHYAR, Dane. *Rhythm of Wholeness*. Wheaton, Illinois: Theosophical Publishing House, 1983.

RUSSELL, Edward W. *Design For Destiny*. New York: Ballentine Books, 1973.

ROBBINS, John. *May All Be Fed: Diet For A New World*. New York: William Morrow, 1992.

ROSSI, Ernest L. *The Psychobiology of Mind-Body Healing*. New York: W.W. Norton, 1986.

SALMON, J. Warren. (ed.). *Alternative Medicines: Popular and Policy Perspectives*. London: Tavistock, 1984.

SELYE, Hans. *The Stress of Life*. New York: McGraw-Hill, 1956.

SHEALY, C. Norman and Myss, Carol M. *The Creation of Health*. Walpole, NH: Stillpoint, 1988.

SIEGEL, Bernard S. *Love, Medicine, and Miracles*. New York: Harper & Row, 1977.

SIMONTON, O. Carl, Matthews-Simonton, Stephanie, and Creighton, James L. *Getting Well Again*. New York: Bantam, 1980.

SOLOMON, George F. "Psychoneuroimmunology: Interactions Between Central Nervous System and Immune System," *Journal of Neuroscience Research*, Vol. 18, No. 1, 1987, p. 1–9.

SPERRY, Roger. "Changing Priorities," *Annual Review of Neuroscience*, 1981, p. 4.

STORR, Anthony. *Solitude*. New York: Ballentine, 1988.

SWAMI RAMA. *A Practical Guide to Holistic Health*, Honesdale, PA: Himalayan Institute, 1979.

_____. *Living with the Himalayan Masters*. Honesdale, PA: Himalayan Institute, 1978.

_____. *Meditation and Its Practice*. Honesdale, PA: Himalayan Institute, 1992.

_____. *Lectures on Yoga*. Honesdale, PA: Himalayan Institute, 1979.

_____. *Science of Breath*. Honesdale, PA: Himalayan Institute, 1998.

TOMPKINS, Peter and Bird, Christopher. *Secrets of the Soil*. New York: Harper & Row, 1989.

VAN DER POST, Laurens. "The Creative Pattern in Primitive Africa," *Eranos Lectures Series*, No. 5. Dallas, TX: Spring Publications, undated.

WEIL, Andrew. *Health and Healing: Understanding Conventional and Alternative Medicine*. Boston: Houghton Mifflin, 1983.

_____. *Spontaneous Healing: How to Discover and Enhance Your Body's Natural Ability to Maintain and Heal Itself*. New York: Knopf, 1995.

WHITE, John and Krippner, Stanley. *Future Science*. New York: Doubleday, 1977.

Index

ABOUT THE AUTHOR

Justin O'Brien, Ph.D. is a pioneer in the exploration of wellness and consciousness. He is known internationally for his programs in individual and corporate wellness. Former Senior Research Fellow in Holistic Medicine at the University of London Medical School, Director of Education and Stress Management at London's Marylebone Health Clinic, Graduate School Director and faculty of the Himalayan International Institute of Yoga Science and Philosophy, he is now faculty at the Alpha Institute of Learning and Spirituality, the University of St. Mary, the University of St. Thomas, and a Founding Board Member of the international Institute of the Himalayan Tradition.

A design consultant for world conferences on health and spirituality in Tokyo, Katmandu, New Delhi, and the United States, he is a gifted speaker and presenter. His global travels have enabled him to synthesize Western and Eastern concepts into a holistic framework for evolving human nature and its behavioral possibilities to higher levels of performance.

O'Brien holds a Doctoral degree in the Philosophy of Consciousness and a Doctorandus degree in Theology from Nijmegen University in the Netherlands, Master of Arts degrees in Philosophy and Religious Studies from Marquette University and St. Albert's College in Oakland, California, and undergraduate degrees in the Classics from the University of Notre Dame and in Philosophy from St. Albert's College. He also holds certification in Ericksonian hypnotherapy from the American Hypnosis Training Academy.

Dr. O'Brien is author of several books in the areas of consciousness and personal development including *Walking with a Himalayan Master*, *The Wellness Tree*, *Running and Breathing*, *A Meeting of Mystic Paths: Christianity and Yoga*, and *Mirrors for Men*.

PUBLICATIONS BY JUSTIN O'BRIEN

The Wellness Tree Audio Tapes

The self-care exercises following selected chapters in this book have been collected into an album of three training cassette tapes led by Dr. Justin O'Brien. The tapes guide you step-by-step through progressive relaxation, tension/relaxation, four breathing practices, hatha yoga postures, the get-to-sleep exercise, meditation, and the sixty-one point exercise. Three tapes in album.

Books

Walking with a Himalayan Master: An American's Odyssey
A Meeting of Mystic Paths: Yoga and Christianity
Mirrors for Men: Daily Reflection
Running and Breathing

Audio Courses

A Life in Harmony: Introduction to Holistic Spirituality
The Art of Stillness: Meditation for Christians
Transforming the Self: Techniques for Personal Development
Sleepless Sleep: The Ancient Art of Conscious Rest
The Wonder of Living
All of the above are four tapes in an album.

Single Audio Tapes

Progressive Relaxation
Breathing I
Meditation
Creativity and the 61 Points
Stretching for Life
Strive Without Stress I
Strive Without Stress II
Get to Sleep!
Intermediate Breathing

To order any of the above items, plus more, including neti pots, call or write to:

Yes International Publishers
1317 Summit Avenue, St. Paul, MN 55105
651-645-6808 / 800-431-1579

www.yespublishers.com
email: yes@yespublishers.com